— A GUIDE FOR —

People Living
with ALS

KRISTEN MASON

Library of Congress Control Number: 2025915058

Book cover design by 100 Covers.

ISBN 978-1-968987-04-6 (paperback)   ISBN 978-1-968987-05-3 (hardcover)
ISBN 978-1-968987-06-0 (ebook)   ISBN 978-1-968987-07-7 (audio)

First Edition Book, August 2025

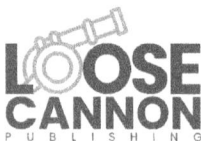

To Brian, my best friend and a true ALS Warrior that without his heroism, courage and "MacGyver®-like" ways this guide would not be possible.

Table of Contents

Prologue

AFTER EXPERIENCING SYMPTOMS for many months, a long-time friend was diagnosed with ALS, a fatal disease, at age 47. A devastating diagnosis at any age, ALS is life changing. The disease progresses at a different rate in each person, and there is no set time at which it will affect any area of the body.

Since ALS is a disease of the nervous system, affecting nerve cells in the brain and spinal cord, there is a loss of muscle control. Those with ALS are stripped of all independence, things that many take for granted each day; scratching an itch, dressing, driving, walking, hugging a friend or loved one…absolutely everything!

As you may already know or will soon find out, ALS is an expensive disease. One wish of my friend was to stay in his home until he passed. That decision seemed fairly simple; however, one big element was missing in that decision. Who would be his caregiver, since he did not have enough resources to pay a professional and no family lived in the area.

His disease was progressing rapidly, so the need for a caregiver was not very far in the future. Many agencies were contacted, but none were affordable. He was running out of time where he might be able to survive alone, so I found myself moving across the country to help him out.

I had never been a caregiver, knew little about it and had a very weak stomach to boot! But it's amazing how quickly something can be learned and how naturally things just flow when needed. Some days things were so busy that I didn't have time to have a weak stomach and quickly got past all of that.

We received consistent praise from therapists and medical personnel on workarounds and how well cared for he was. I credit all of that to my friend. He was a very creative, innovative and talented person who did everything quickly and extremely well. He knew what he wanted and was always extremely grateful and kind, never getting upset about anything and always coaching me through it. I learned a lot while caring for him.

A few months before he passed, he told me that once everything was over, he wanted me to write a guide to help others living with ALS. I hope you will find this information helpful and that it will make your journey through this condition—whether as a patient or as a caregiver—a little easier.

Chapter 1

Introduction

SPRING HAS SPRUNG, the birds are singing, and some rough months are behind you. You're still feeling a lot of stress from the previous months, but things are looking up. After all, winter is past and your favorite season is here, saying it's time to dust off the golf clubs, break out your bathing suit and start planning your next trip to a tropical paradise.

The days go by, and everything seems the same as it was the previous year. You're still going to work, spending time with family and friends, and doing activities you enjoy. As the summer draws near, you start to notice a little change in your speech. You can detect slurring in your words, though no one has said anything to you. Is it just your imagination? After all, you have been very stressed and a little tired lately.

You communicate a lot, but speaking is becoming very exhausting. It feels like you can no longer control your tongue the way you once could or form words in the same way. Maybe it is time to see a doctor. You make an appointment and get a full physical, only for the doctor to put you on some medication for your speech and refer you to a therapist. You know you feel different than what was once your norm, but no one else notices. Why are you being referred to a therapist? Again, you wonder if you are just imagining the impaired speech pattern.

Months pass, and by now you have visited several more doctors, only to be poked and prodded many times with no resolution. Your speech seems to be getting worse, and now some people are even beginning to point it out. Some are asking if you have an alcohol problem.

Summer is now in all its glory, and it is time to fire up the smoker and the barbeque. You just did some grocery shopping and got the best rack of beef ribs money could buy. Like always, you try to be as efficient as possible and grab all the bags of groceries out of your truck at the same time, so you only have to make one trip. You're almost at the kitchen when your right hand gives way, and all the bags fall to the floor. What in the world is going on! You gather the scattered groceries and eventually manage to lug everything to the kitchen counter.

Your arm feels a little weaker than usual, but you're still able to muddle through and get the meat and sides prepared. The day was wonderful with family and friends, and yet you can't help but focus on the changes happening in your body.

Another week passes, and you're just days away from heading to the Emerald Coast for what will presumably be a period of some much-needed rest and recuperation. Maybe sprawling on the beach for a week and listening to the softly crashing waves will help your body rejuvenate.

Departure day is finally here. You quickly pack your suitcase and drive to the airport. Your carry-on luggage is small but seems to be harder than usual to hoist into the overhead bin. It is a struggle, but you get it done. A short time later, you land at the airport, and now even raising your arm high enough to pull down your carry-on luggage is almost a challenge. You are not comfortable driving the rental car, so you have your companion do all the driving. You finally arrive at your digs for the week. It looks just perfect, a peaceful place where you can relax when you're not stretched out on the sand.

The first order of business, before invading the sand, is to head to the grocery store. Cooking is a huge part of your life, and just because you are on vacation there is no reason not to cook. You get all the groceries you will need for the next week and head back to your rental. You pack a few snacks and you're off to the beach.

After a relaxing afternoon on the sand and surf, you start dinner. When trying to carry the frying pan over to the sink to add a little water, your hand again gives way. You do your best to let the pan down easily to the floor but still spill some meat. Something is going on with your right hand; it's just not working like it used to. The hand seems to be bending okay, but the strength it once had is no longer there.

You had an enjoyable week at the beach but couldn't do a lot of exploring on foot. Your feet were shuffling a bit, and walking too far was tiring and difficult. It is time to head back to the airport, and although the flight home is short, the very thought of waiting at the airport for the plane to take off is exhausting; you've just not been yourself lately. When it came time to put your carry-on luggage in the overhead compartment, it was a struggle to lift it high enough. How could this be? You just put the same luggage in the overhead bin, six days prior. Now your companion had to help you lift your luggage, and you returned home.

Your symptoms didn't dissipate from the week of rest and relaxation as you had hoped. You started thinking that, based on your symptoms, you may have Amyotrophic Lateral Sclerosis (ALS). You made an appointment with your primary care doctor and shared your concern. The doctor's response was that you could not have ALS, because none of her other patients have ever had ALS. The doctor discounted your concern and ran a series of blood tests for other diseases, including Wilson's Disease. All tests came back negative, so the doctor told you there was nothing further she could do, and you could work with a neurologist as a next step. The problem with that was that you would have to wait another three months before you could see a neurologist. The months seemed long as you waited for your appointment; meanwhile, your speech seemed to be getting worse.

The day is finally here for your appointment, and the neurologist is very concerned that you may have ALS, based on your speech patterns and the muscle weakness in your right arm, hand and tongue. You are sent for more blood tests, along with magnetic resonance imaging (MRI) of the spine and electromyography (EMG) to measure the electrical activity of the muscles and nerves.

The neurologist has not discussed any results yet, and the results that are coming in electronically are causing even more concern. You check online to see what some of the results from the blood test and MRI may mean, and you are now certain that you have a serious condition.

You go to your last appointment for now, the EMG, and it is time to hear your fate. The neurologist says there is a 99 percent probability that it is ALS, based on the symptoms and results. The diagnosis can never be 100 percent accurate with ALS. It is the news that you dreaded most. You have ALS, bulbar onset ALS to be exact, and you are told that you have one to four years left on this Earth.

Chapter 2

Diagnosis . . . Now What?

NOW THAT YOU have been diagnosed with ALS, life will never be the same again. You must completely shift gears and change course, putting aside the long-term goals you once had. Maybe you can revisit those goals in the future; you're not ready to throw in the towel to this disease just yet. While still mentally processing the information that you were given earlier, you notify a few family members and friends. It is overwhelming and exhausting trying to explain what ALS is, as most individuals will have no idea.

So many things are running through your head, a myriad of things on your bucket list to complete and so many affairs to be put in order as soon as possible. Gosh…where to start?

You decide that one of your biggest priorities is ensuring that your assets are distributed per your wishes, upon your death. You do not yet have a last will and testament, living will or a trust in place, so you contact a trust attorney and get the first available appointment. Before your appointment, you brainstorm about all your assets to make the meeting as purposeful as possible. Some of the information to gather is as follows:

- Bank account(s), including financial institution name(s) and account number(s)
- Investments, including financial institution name(s) and account number(s), e.g., stocks, mutual funds, bonds, certificates of deposit

- Real property, including address(es) and parcel number(s)
- Vehicle title(s)

Some other items to consider are as follows:

- Individual(s) who will hold Power of Attorney
- Individual(s) who will be your personal representative(s), responsible for managing your estate after you pass
- Individual(s) or organization(s) to which your assets will be left (beneficiaries)
- Guardian(s) for any minor children
- Funeral arrangements, celebration of life, burial and/or cremation instructions

There may come a time when you are unable to communicate your healthcare wishes. If these are documented in your living will, there will be no question about what healthcare measures should be taken or any that should be avoided. Some things to consider are as follows:

- Wishes regarding hospitalization
- Decisions regarding palliative care or hospice care
- Staying in your home or going to in-patient care

The day of your appointment arrives, and you discuss everything with the attorney. The attorney gets all that noted and is ready to work on the will and trust. A couple of weeks later, everything is documented in writing and ready for you to sign. The attorney makes certain that you are aware that an amendment can be made to the document if anything changes in the future. What a relief it will be, getting this done and knowing that you can add or change anything down the road, if needed.

Depending on disease progression and one's ability to work, contacting Medicare may be another priority for individuals who reside in the United States of America (United States). If an individual qualifies, Medicare will assist in setting up medical insurance, monthly payments to the individual and potentially monthly payments to minor children until the age of 18.

Some individuals may choose to also obtain a supplemental insurance policy outside of Medicare. Every individual must explore the options that are best for them. If eligible and moving forward with Medicare, the two parts that seem to be most beneficial to those with ALS are Medicare Part A and Part B for inpatient and outpatient care.

Some prescriptions required for the care of those with ALS are quite costly. Medicare Part D may be the best option for drug coverage for those who qualify; however, each individual must weigh the options on what may be most cost-effective for them. An additional policy may be worth exploring to compare and contrast the costs, including many of the discounted prescription programs seen online or on television.

Two of the items that were weighing heavily on you are now in process. You'd like to start focusing on your bucket list while you are able to, but must keep in mind that you still have no definitive plan moving forward from the neurologist. What are some of the items on your bucket list, and do you need to speak to the neurologist before performing any of them? Which are the most feasible and most important to you? Traveling to a different country? Completing a work of art? Skydiving? Ziplining? Taking a cruise? Deep sea fishing? Flyfishing? Hunting? Which item will you schedule first? Will you be able to complete more than one item on your bucket list?

Many of your friends and family are requesting to spend time with you, so you must decide who will be invited along on your bucket list adventure(s). In addition, checking with the neurologist to ensure you are clear to travel and/or complete your adventures is advisable. It may be a good idea to request a medical note from the neurologist, which can be presented to available medical personnel in case of emergency while you are traveling or otherwise away from home.

While working through all of this, you again realize that the neurologist sent you on your way with no direction and no future appointments. You have heard that some cases of ALS are associated with certain genes. Should you inquire about genetic testing? The answer is yes! Not only will this help to confirm your diagnosis, if you have one of the associated genes, certain medications target one of the more common genes. In addition, there are clinical trials that focus on certain genes as well. While there is no cure as of this writing, it is thought that certain medications may help slow the progression of the disease in some individuals. Taking medications is a personal choice and something that should be discussed with medical professionals so you can make the right decision.

Chapter 3

Being Proactive!

THE FOLLOWING INFORMATION is designed to assist people living with ALS (pALS) and caregivers (cALS) to make daily life a little more manageable. As the disease progresses differently for everyone, not everything in this guide may work for all pALS, and what may work one day may not work the next. There is one major takeaway in this guide that cannot be emphasized enough. It is that you must be proactive regarding your own health and the many devices required to make pALS able to function in day-to-day living. Do not wait until something is needed to try and get it, because at that point it is too late! Getting items cleared through insurance is generally not a fast process. Having doctors, neurologists, therapists, etc., draw up paperwork and sign off on something is not quick either. Those two factors combined can take several months before you receive the equipment, even assuming that it is approved after all the waiting.

As you read through this guide, let it provoke thought on what may make everyday life easier, with a disease that has no boundaries. ALS is a very expensive disease, and not everyone can afford all the devices, medications or supplies necessary. That is where some creative workarounds may have to come into play. Certain ALS organizations also allow assistive equipment to be borrowed or provide financial assistance to purchase equipment. Some of those organizations are covered in Chapter 17.

As the disease progresses, different supplies and equipment will be needed at different stages. Some things will continue to be used, while others will be phased out and new items introduced. Some items may take more time or resources to procure than others and may or may not be covered by insurance.

Some of these items are discussed in the guide, with notes indicating whether they worked for us or did not work at all. While symptoms may vary between individuals, for clarity in this guide, please consider the following as a general guideline for the stages of ALS:

- **Early-Stage:** Muscle weakness, slurred speech, and the ability to perform daily tasks in a modified and/or slower manner.

- **Middle-Stage:** Increased mobility challenges, requiring use of assistive devices such as a rollator or Hoyer lift, insertion of feeding tube.

- **Late-Stage:** Inability to communicate verbally without assistive device, reliance on nutrition via a feeding tube only, limited muscle control, pain, anxiety, claustrophobia.

- **End-Stage:** Focus on palliative and/or hospice care, respiratory complications, heightened pain, anxiety, claustrophobia.

These examples reflect our specific experience. Although this guide is based on caring for a male pALS and some items may seem tailored to his needs, there are equivalent alternatives for others—for example, swapping a facial razor for a leg razor.

Chapter 4

Transportation

TRANSPORTATION IS A major component that may become difficult early on, depending on whether you own a vehicle and the type of vehicle you own. Our transportation was a raised truck, which became increasingly difficult to get in and out of, especially when a rollator became essential. Eventually, to get to appointments, it became necessary to rent a sport utility vehicle (SUV) that was high enough for the pALS to easily get in and out of and also allowed enough legroom to easily swing his legs around. The rental vehicle was a substantial expense, until the truck could be sold and an accessible vehicle within budget could be located and purchased.

Handicapped Placard

Although the pALS may be mobile and possibly still driving, it is not too early to begin thinking about applying for a "handicapped" placard or "permanently disabled" license plates. The application process begins with the neurologist and must be submitted and processed by the local driving bureau. Even if it seems like it is not needed at the time, there will come a time when it becomes indispensable. Remember, be proactive. It is better to apply for and receive the placard or license plates early than not have them when required.

Vehicle and Transportation

It is not too early to consider this significant issue potentially involving a major purchase. Initially, the pALS will likely be required to attend medical appointments in person and will need transportation to get to those appointments, an ALS clinic or other outings. While the pALS is more mobile, there may be no issue with transportation in a regular vehicle. Some areas may even have public transportation or a dial-a-ride type service that can transport pALS, while others do not have that resource. As the disease progresses, and it becomes difficult, if not impossible, for the pALS to get into a regular vehicle, an accessible vehicle will become an option to be considered. Vehicles with conversions that allow wheelchairs to enter are generally more costly than vehicles with no conversion. This is something that should be researched sooner rather than later, so that a vehicle that is within a specific price range can be purchased when appropriate.

When researching vehicles, ensure that pALS are involved in the type of vehicle(s) being explored. The disease is already hard, and some pALS indicate not wanting to be transported in the typical minivan conversion. As technology has progressed, several other types of conversions have become available, including trucks and SUVs.

Aside from the type of vehicle, other factors should also be taken into consideration while conducting research, such as:

- the length and height of the pALS in their wheelchair
- ramp position
- manual ramp versus power ramp and weight capacity
- position where the pALS will sit in the vehicle
- conversion manufacturer and service centers

The size and especially height of the pALS while sitting in their wheelchair is extremely important. Vehicles are not one-size-fits-all, and the roof height may be too low to accommodate some pALS. In addition, there may not be enough legroom to accommodate the wheelchair, footplates or the overhang of the pALS' feet on the footplates of a wheelchair. Another consideration is the amount of room required to allow rotation of the wheelchair in the vehicle, if needed, to properly position the wheelchair for transport.

Note: If you want to ensure extra headroom, a large entry door height, wider door width and ramp, the Chevy Traverse provides some of the largest dimensions in all these aspects in the industry, as of this writing. The ramp will vary depending on which company does the conversion. This is the vehicle that worked best for us all around. A minivan was not desirable, and like in some sport utility vehicles, it was difficult to manipulate a large electric wheelchair and still provide enough space for a person 6 feet 4 inches tall.

The position where the ramp is located on the vehicle is another important factor. Generally, there are two possible positions: either a side entry that is curbside or a rear entry. While determining the best position for your application, think about places where you may be parking at medical appointments or other places, along with traffic patterns. Which will be safer for the person operating the ramp as well as the pALS regarding entering or exiting from the vehicle, keeping in mind there may be cross traffic in the area? The position of the ramp also affects the interior of the vehicle regarding additional seating and additional room for turning. In some vehicles, whether the front passenger seat can be removed to accommodate a wheelchair position can also be a relevant consideration.

Ramps come with either manual or power operation. When determining which is best for you, try to consider all factors. There are obviously pros and cons for both. One major difference is the cost and maintenance. As you may guess, a power ramp is more expensive and requires regular maintenance to ensure it is functioning properly and continues functioning. The power ramp is more convenient, especially when trying to juggle the many things you are likely to be carrying when leaving the house. The power operation just requires the push of a button with a finger to open and close, and nothing more than that. Many power ramps stow out of the way of all passengers. Manual operation requires more physical work. The ramps are fairly lightweight and generally not too difficult to deploy or fold up. The manual ramps usually fold and are stored in an upright position, just inside the door. Speaking of weight, it is advisable to double-check the weight capacity of the ramp. Theoretically, all ramps should be able to accommodate pALS and wheelchairs, but that is not something you should assume, as power wheelchairs are very heavy.

Note: Power worked best for us; however, the very last time we used the vehicle, the door would not activate to allow the ramp to deploy. However, a manual release was installed in the rear of the vehicle with the conversion, so we were still able to get the door open, ramp down and back up to load up. The door started functioning again on the next use, and we were able to easily exit the vehicle. We did have the opportunity to use a manual ramp while on vacation for one week, and it was significantly more difficult for the operator of the ramp. It continued to become detached from the vehicle and did not feel sturdy when the wheelchair was on it. This may not be the case with all manual ramps; it is simply an observation regarding the ramp on the rental vehicle we used.

If you are researching vehicles early, all of this may be hard to picture, and it may be difficult to decide, especially if the pALS does not yet have, or has not yet been measured for, a wheelchair. You may wonder why it matters where the pALS will be sitting in the vehicle. This is important because different vehicles have different roof and door heights, which impact both ingress and egress. It is also worth noting, especially if the pALS desires to sit in the front passenger seat position, that some manufacturers slant the roof of the vehicle before the windshield starts to slant, so the roof height in the front position may be even lower than the roof height at a different position in the vehicle. You also want to determine if the plan is to have the pALS face the front or side of the vehicle and if there is space for them to turn around once inside the vehicle. Will the wheelchair have to be backed in to get into the proper position? Pulled in forward? How will the pALS exit?

There are several conversion companies located in the United States; two of the commonly heard ones are BraunAbility® (Braun) and ATC Distributors, LLC® (ATC). A notable difference between the two companies' products is the ramp style. Braun has a long ramp that protrudes beyond the bodyline of the vehicle when deployed. ATC provides a ramp similar to the one used by Braun, as well as a ramp integrated into the vehicle. The side door features a gull-wing design, opening upward with hinges at the top, while part of the floor of the vehicle drops straight down to the ground, creating the ramp. The power ATC ramp is what we had and what worked best for us. One significant benefit of this type of ramp is that a wheelchair can easily go up and down the ramp without risk of driving off the edge, whereas a notable drawback is ensuring there is van accessible space so that the door has room to go up to release the ramp. In addition, there is added road noise inside the vehicle while driving, from having the vehicle's floor modified. While one of the ramp styles may be more appealing than the other, perhaps the best place to start is by calling both manufacturers to determine if a service center is present near your residence. This is important in case the ramp needs servicing or a preventative maintenance check-up to ensure it is in tip-top shape. Depending on the location of the service centers, you could make the decision on which style and manufacturer will be best.

The conversion vehicles that accommodate wheelchairs tend to be considerably more expensive than other vehicles, so you may really have to shop around to find one within your price point. In addition, if you find one out of state that checks all the boxes, keep in mind that you do not necessarily have to go to the location to view it. A third party can be hired to view and inspect the vehicle, or the buyer can request that the seller take it to the nearest dealership for inspection. The buyer will likely have to pay the cost of the inspection, but it is well worth the money, not to mention peace of mind. If it all checks out, the vehicle can be shipped to you.

Chapter 5

Supplies and Modifications

As mentioned previously, ALS progresses differently in individuals. The supplies mentioned in this section may be needed at short notice by some pALS and quite a bit farther down the line by others. Please also note that this guide does not mention all the items available; it just touches upon items of which the author has experience or knowledge. Everything that is typically needed for each day will be identified in the remaining sections. Hopefully, this will assist in putting some things on your radar and perhaps introduce some items that you haven't thought you may require. It will also allow time to borrow the item(s) from an ALS organization's loan closet, apply for a grant through an ALS organization, or speak to one of the pALS' therapists or the neurologist about obtaining the item through insurance.

Alarm

An alarm clock of some sort, whether it is on a cell phone or elsewhere, is vital to keep things on schedule, be it medications, range of motion exercises, oxygen check, standing to stretch or standing to avoid pressure wounds. It will be useful at all stages of ALS.

Allen Wrench Set

Both a standard and metric Allen wrench set are recommended if an electric wheelchair is going to be utilized. Adjustments will undoubtedly need to be made; besides, not all screws are the same size. A cushioned grip hex t-handle set works very well, allowing for some leverage while turning the screws.

Alternating Air Pressure Mattress Pad

A physical therapist recommended that we purchase this, believing it would assist with sleeping during middle-stage ALS. It is intended for a hospital bed, so it comes in twin size. The pressure can be adjusted from light to maximum. When it was first removed from the box, it was tried in the lift recliner to see if the oscillating air pressure would help relieve any of the pain from sitting. It did not oscillate properly in the chair since the chair wasn't flat, so that was not an option. It was then placed on the bed and inflated to the lowest pressure. The pALS was placed on the mattress pad, but found it extremely hard. There was no way the pALS could sleep on it, so it was boxed up and returned.

Augmentative and Alternative Communication (AAC) Device

Going back to being proactive, this is something to discuss with the speech therapist earlier rather than later. Speech is going to become difficult, if not non-existent. The pALS' ability to use their hands will diminish. In order to communicate, they will need some sort of device. In our case, the pALS used a Tobii Dynavox®, which was an amazing lifesaver. It is an iPadOS® with eye-controlled technology; it was the central command center of the house. The pALS could text, call, email, speak with others in the room, use all necessary applications (apps) and websites for daily business, play games, and control the television and indoor climate. The pALS had this in place many months before it was needed full-time, which allowed him to get accustomed to using his eyes to communicate even before he was in a situation where he absolutely needed it and could not function without it.

Note: When researching, decide if the pALS will be communicating more with those who have Android™ or Apple™ devices. The pALS in our case got the TD Pilot™ option, which was fantastic. The only drawback was that anyone with an Android device could not text the pALS, as his device only supported iMessage®, so any message sent with an Android device could only be sent to the pALS' cell phone.

Additional considerations:

- *Try to determine whether or not the pALS will be utilizing Ability Drive™ now or in the future. More about this can be found in this chapter under, "Wheelchair, Electric".*

- *Voice banking may be something to contemplate; however, the pALS had someone with a similar voice do the voice banking for his device and it sounded very robotic. After paying the money for it, the pALS ended up using one of the voices included with the AAC. Since that time, artificial intelligence (AI) has been tested and appears to be superior to the traditional voice banking used by the pALS, if feasible.*

Augmentative and Alternative Communication (AAC) Stand

To ensure that the Tobii Dynavox was readily available for the pALS while in the lift recliner, a floating floor mount by ConnectIT™ was purchased. The stand contains four locking wheels, enabling it to either stay in place or be easily moved, as required.

There are similar mounts by various manufacturers that can be attached to an electric wheelchair to enable the pALS to always have the AAC available.

Back Scratcher

A back scratcher is a way to assist pALS in reaching an itch when mobility is changing. The pALS had a metal adjustable back scratcher that could be extended a little over 24 inches and a stationary wood one that is about 18 inches and a little larger in girth than the adjustable one. Both were used in early-stage and early middle-stage ALS. The adjustable one was used as a head/scalp massager from middle- to end-stage ALS to help relax the pALS.

Bilevel Positive Airway Pressure (BiPAP®)

A BiPAP machine may be needed at some point to be worn while sleeping, resting or around the clock. A tight seal must be maintained around the mask. There are various masks that can be tried; we had them all. The BiPAP may take some getting used to for some pALS and may have to be used a few minutes or hours per day, here and there, to get adjusted to it before trying to sleep with it in place.

Note: The pALS tried a BiPAP during middle-stage ALS and had an extremely hard time getting used to it, due to claustrophobia as well as just having something on his face while sleeping. The pALS was accustomed to side sleeping and now had to be a back sleeper. We had the BiPAP for three months, and about one month in, the pALS went from using it for about two minutes per day to sleeping with it for ten hours per night…for four nights. After that, the pALS determined the claustrophobia had come back, and we eventually ended up returning the machine to the company.

BOTOX®

Some neurologists recommend injecting BOTOX into the salivary glands to retard saliva production. The pALS first attempted this in middle-stage ALS when saliva was increasing. At that point, the pALS was still able to swallow the saliva without using a suction device. About one week after the injections, however, saliva increased substantially, and a suction device was needed. The neurologist only used about 50 percent of the dose since it was the first time, so the pALS tried again three months later—now in late-stage ALS. Saliva had been out of control for the preceding two months. About two weeks after the second set of injections, the pALS got one day of dry mouth, and then the saliva went back to being out of control; out of control meaning suctioning every one to two minutes. I recommend researching before using this method to find what is right for the pALS. Aside from many medications that are made to assist with saliva, there have also been some other techniques recently unveiled that may assist with slowing saliva. Other surgical options were also explored;

however, the pALS decided not to move forward with any of them since he was in late-stage ALS.

Carpe® Antiperspirant Hand Lotion

As the pALS loses the ability to move and straighten the fingers, the hands tend to sweat more and may develop an odor. This lotion was a huge help in assisting in drying out the hands and eliminating odor. It was especially helpful when wearing hand braces, since the hands would get hot on the fabric in the warmer months. We used the original scent, which only had a mild essence, middle- through end-stage ALS.

Catheter

The pALS did not want a catheter, as most people may not. A medication was available for males, in this case, that enabled the pALS not to have a catheter. The medication, Tamsulosin, could not be crushed and put down a feeding tube. A suspension formula was created at the compounding pharmacy to enable it to be administered through the feeding tube. Speak to a urologist to see what is right for the pALS; however, most urologists will likely do whatever is possible for the pALS to keep them catheter-free, since catheters come with a whole other set of problems.

Note: The pALS had an overnight stay in the hospital during late-stage ALS and wanted to keep the catheter in and try it out at home to see if it made things easier for him. We found ourselves in the emergency room the next night, having it removed, as the pALS decided for certain he did not want one, and the medication was working for him.

Clothing

Beginning in early-stage ALS, dressing will get progressively harder for the pALS. Buttoning and snapping may eventually become too difficult. To keep the pALS dressing/undressing themselves for as long as possible, pants or shorts with an elastic waist will help. Some companies make nice-looking elastic-waisted garments for pALS who do not necessarily want to wear joggers or sweat-type pants. As the disease progresses and the pALS requires assistance to dress, the elastic waist bottoms can still be used, as they make it easier for the cALS to put on and pull up. Thinner material shirts with a little stretch also will help the pALS to dress themselves, as well as make it easier for the cALS when assisting. The thinner shirts are also quite helpful as the pALS becomes progressively more immobile, considering that a thinner shirt is not as hot when sitting in a wheelchair or lift recliner.

There is also "adaptive" clothing available. This is clothing that comes apart and can be put in place with Velcro closures or snaps at the seams. The clothing can be put on in two pieces or opened in certain areas to make it easier to slip on. Something that would be more cost effective is to buy Velcro, split the pALS' existing clothing up the seams, sew the Velcro in and make your own adaptive clothing. This method requires a little work; however, it will cut back on the expense of purchasing a new wardrobe and may help the pALS to feel more comfortable wearing their "normal" clothes. For the pALS, we utilized elastic waistbands and thin material shirts during the day and a lightweight tech stretch fabric tank top for sleeping.

Note: When dressing the pALS or if the pALS is self-dressing, put arms into the shirt before pulling it over the head, and while removing, follow the reverse order. This will help with the dressing and also not cause any undue pain to the shoulders or neck.

Cooling Vest

It is so important that a pALS does not get overheated, and sitting in a wheelchair, unable to move much, if at all, is very hot. In our case, the pALS researched this extensively and found the best option to be a cooling vest made by Glacier Tek™ that cools to 59°F for about 150 minutes. The vest has ice packs that are easy to insert and Velcro on the shoulders, making it easy to adjust and slip over the head of the pALS, so that it can be strapped around the waist. A cooling vest is highly recommended, especially for those who live in warmer climates. It made the difference of being able to go outside versus staying indoors all day during the summer months. It was also useful for medical appointments in the summer months, since sitting in the wheelchair was so hot.

Cough Assist

The pALS was getting phlegm, causing a lot of coughing when eating and drinking, which provoked the urge to quit both essential activities; the hours of coughing were not worth it. Two months after the pALS quit eating and drinking orally, in middle-stage ALS, a medical professional suggested to the pALS that a cough assist would enable oral intake of food and drink. The cough assist would make the phlegm come up easily and also strengthen the diaphragm if used daily. The pALS agreed to try. One small spoonful of applesauce was attempted, and the pALS immediately got phlegm. Despite attempting over twenty rounds of the cough assist, the secretion never came up freely. The cough assist was tried again on a few occasions with the same result. This was just our experience with it; others may have a different experience. The cough assist was returned to the company.

Note: If the cough assist really does strengthen the diaphragm, it may be beneficial to be proactive and use it daily to assist with coughing, in the event the pALS gets pneumonia or some similar condition. That way, there is more strength in the diaphragm for the pALS to get the "junk" out of the lungs; we found this to be a struggle for the pALS in late-stage ALS.

Crocs™ Classic All-Terrain Sandals

These are adjustable sandals with a rugged sole and two upper straps. They provide stability for a pALS for use as water shoes in the swimming pool, walking across sand at the beach or just walking around the house. These were utilized in early- and middle-stage ALS when the pALS was still mobile.

Doorstop – Kickdown

If the residence has any doors that do not stay open without someone holding the door, a one-touch kickdown doorstop works really well. This will come in especially helpful when trying to get a wheelchair through the door. It comes equipped with a lever to step on when ready to close the door, so it is all hands-free.

Note: We took the wheelchair out the side door to the garage for ease, and the door stopper was extremely helpful. It is hard to hold the door with a foot or hand while holding other items and trying to assist the pALS to get the wheelchair through the door and down the ramp.

Electric Earwax Removal Tool

An ear irrigation flushing system, ear cleaner and camera were used when the cALS first came on as the pALS had been unable to properly groom his ears for months, and the wax was very impacted. The camera was helpful to see trouble areas. Once the ears were cleaned, they were maintained with cotton swabs.

Note: Our experience down the line was that ears that are too clean cause a deep itch in the ear canal. Being mindful of that, the outsides of the ears were washed and cleaned daily. The insides were examined daily and cleaned as needed, leaving them slightly dirty. If cleaned too much and itching occurs, rubbing a small amount of Cortizone-10® in front of the ear and on the tragus (flap) will help stop the itching.

Eyedrops

Drops may be needed to lubricate the eyes, especially if using an eye-tracking device. We used gel drops throughout the day on most days, from middle-stage through end-stage ALS.

Note: If using an eye tracking device, excessive redness in one or both eyes may require a visit with an eye doctor, as there may be inflammation.

Eyeglasses/Sunglasses Neck Cord

A neck cord can assist pALS in keeping their eyeglasses close and prevent these from falling to the floor in early- and middle-stage ALS. Once the pALS could no longer put on his eyeglasses, the cord was removed, and the cALS would put the glasses on and take them off.

Facial Tissues

We purchased facial tissues by the case, due to the pALS' high volume of nasal secretions, during early- and middle-stage ALS. The nasal secretions were most pronounced in the morning and while eating. We primarily used Kleenex® with lotion. In middle-stage ALS, the pALS underwent a posterior nasal nerve ablation, which significantly reduced the nasal secretions.

Finger Splint

Made to support two or three fingers, this device splints the fingers and straightens the knuckles and can be used on either hand. This was utilized in early-stage ALS when the fingers were beginning to curl. It assists with holding the fingers straight and helps to relieve some of the pain caused by curling fingers. It is difficult to put on without assistance as it also straps around the forearm, but it can be done. The best approach is to have someone else get it set up for the pALS so that the hand can be slipped in and out, and the strap just has to be tightened to put on or loosened to remove the splint.

Gait Belt

A gait belt measures 2 inches wide, has a metal buckle and is used to assist the pALS to move, such as for standing up and holding the pALS erect while walking. The device makes it easier for pALS by providing support or the extra assistance needed to stand, while putting less pressure on the back of cALS when assisting.

Note: We utilized the gait belt a lot for standing to give the pALS the extra support needed to get out of the sliding shower chair and off the toilet. When the pALS was still standing with the help of the lift recliner, but using the Hoyer lift for transportation, the gait belt was rarely utilized. With the lift recliner, a little assistance from a hand in the pALS' armpit to help him stand was all that was needed.

Hand Splint/Brace

The splints utilized by the pALS were made by Restorative Medical™ and came in a size that was right for the pALS' hands. These splints are soft where the hand touches, but underneath the washable fabric is foam over an aluminum base. The splints can be molded to give the pALS' hands as much support as needed. The splints, or braces as many call them, are very beneficial in making the pALS' hands more pliable and therefore less painful. The pALS could only wear them for a short time, when first received, due to soreness in the hands. Eventually, the pALS wore them overnight in bed. After doing that for a month or so, the pALS decided to wear them only from the time he got up to bedtime, in the hope of getting better sleep without something on his hands. They would be removed and put back on each time he stood up so his hands could rest on the rollator for balance. These devices were utilized from middle- to late-stage ALS. During the latter part of late-stage ALS, the pALS became claustrophobic and unable to tolerate anything on his hands. The hands started to become stiffer, despite doing range of motion exercises daily. Several times, we tried just laying the pALS' hands on the braces, one at a time, and not closing the straps, just to try stretching the fingers out a bit.

Note: Braces tend to make the hands hot, so Carpe was very helpful in controlling the sweat factor of the hands and the smell of the braces. The braces are also washable and dry fastest when clipped on a hanger and hung outdoors.

Head Strap

One thing that was an ongoing battle was the headrest on the electric wheelchair. Nothing seemed to hold the head in place. The head strap on the wheelchair was very poor and uncomfortable. It required a cap to be worn on the head to alleviate some discomfort and to try and keep it in place. An airplane/car head support strap was purchased to try to hold the head in place, as it was touted to help stop one's head from bobbing. It was very soft and comfortable, but the one time it was tried in the car, it was not effective. This was attempted in middle-stage ALS when head control was declining.

Heating Pad/Rice Pack – Large, Microwavable

An unscented, microwavable heating and freezer pack combination, measuring 7 inches by 24 inches, was used to apply heat to the pALS' hips in an attempt to ease the pain. It was placed in the freezer once to try a cold press, but heat proved more effective. This was used in late- and end-stage ALS.

Heating Pad Rice/Bean Pack – Small, Microwavable

An unscented microwavable heating pad with a washable cover, measuring 6 inches by 12 inches, was initially purchased to be used for hip pain; however, the size of the heating pad was a bit too small for it to stay on the hip without falling off. It was covered with a pillowcase and repurposed as what we called the "bag". It was placed on the headrest and used to hold the pALS' head from falling to one side while sitting in the lift recliner. This was used in late- and end-stage ALS.

Heating Pad, Traditional

An electric heating pad with controller to customize heat intensity did not find favor with the pALS, as it was not hot enough. He tried it on a few occasions but always went back to the rice pack.

Heel Elevators

There was a period in middle-stage ALS where the pALS' heels were getting sore, due to sitting more than he had previously done. Many different solutions available on the market were attempted, including two half rounds and a three-quarters round massage table bolster. The half round did not elevate the heels enough, and the three-quarter round was too much. Also attempted were foot support pillows and foot wedge pillows that wrap around the ankles and elevate the heels; neither elevated the heels at all, while still allowing pressure on the heels. We ended up alternating a thin bed pillow and a pillow from the couch for a while and ultimately ended up just using the thin bed pillow. The objective was supposed to be to keep pressure off the heels, but the pALS wanted his heels to lie on the pillow. We managed to avoid pressure wounds, and the soreness subsided. The pillow was used during middle- through end-stage ALS.

Hinges and Doorways

Are the doorways wide enough to allow for a walker, rollator or wheelchair to pass through without making contact? One workaround is to purchase "swing away" or "offset" door hinges. Installation of such hinges allows extra space in the door opening by keeping the door flush with the doorjamb when open, allowing barrier-free access. These hinges may allow just enough space so that no major modifications need to be made to the doorway.

Helpful hints when purchasing:

- order the same size and shape hinge as is currently on the door
- double-check the quantity, as many are sold individually, rather than in a set of three

Note: These hinges were a lifesaver for us. The extra inch or two allowed the wheelchair to easily pass through to get into the bathroom. Prior to this, the wheelchair was being taken as far as possible and then we had to try to traverse the final distance by walking with a rollator, which was very difficult as the disease progressed. These hinges were utilized beginning in middle-stage ALS; however, installing them earlier would have been beneficial.

Hoyer Lift, Electric

An electric Hoyer lift makes things much easier than using a manual Hoyer lift. Many, including the one we utilized, are foldable and portable. Electric Hoyer lifts have definite advantages over manual lifts, including a remote control, and the ability for the legs to be opened wider than the manual lift, allowing it to fit around the lift recliner chair. It also has a longer handle on top, which allows the pALS to get closer to objects or farther into the bed and is able to raise the pALS higher vertically than the manual lift.

Hoyer Lift, Hydraulic (Manual)

This is a robust Hoyer lift and generally the one provided by insurance. It is more difficult to use, as it does not lift as high, making it difficult to get the pALS into bed. In addition, the handle on top is not as long and the legs do not open as wide, so it does not reach around or over a large lift recliner chair. That being said, the pALS cannot be pulled over the chair or object while lowered, as the handle to lower the pALS is on the opposite side of the lift. Therefore, the cALS has to release the handle and try to run around the chair to get the pALS in the right place. Fortunately, the pALS I assisted was proactive and got the lift early through insurance, allowing time to try it before it was needed. Quickly realizing it would not work for the pALS, we contacted the local ALS Association to request an electric lift. They did not have one in the loan closet but generously purchased one for the pALS through a grant.

Leg Braces – Ankle Foot Orthosis (AFOs)

The pALS researched ankle foot braces and was interested in getting one at middle-stage ALS; however, upon hearing the co-pay amount, the pALS opted out on the plea that a brace would likely not help that much, especially with only a limited amount of time left in which he might be able to walk. As such, there is no actual experience to share of using an AFO. However, this device is highlighted here to bring awareness that there is something that may be able to assist in stabilizing weak ankle muscles and help with a drop foot or dragging toes.

Lip Balm

Lip balm was used throughout all stages of ALS and especially during late- and end-stage ALS, as hydration was becoming harder to maintain. Moreover, the constant suctioning of saliva dried out the pALS' lips.

Milk Frother Wand

A handheld battery-operated milk frother wand/small whisk with a stand was a huge timesaver with medications that required mixing with or dissolving in water, vitamins, etc. The device eliminated a lot of stirring with a spoon. The brand that worked for us was *Zulay Executive Series*®.

Neck Brace, Cervical

The cervical collar utilized by the pALS was the *Ossur Miami J*® brand; however, other brands are available too. It helped to hold the neck in place and relieve some of the pain and pressure from deterioration of the spine as well as the neck getting weaker and being harder to hold up. The device was used mostly outside the house for car trips and air travel in early- and up to middle-stage ALS.

Neck Brace, Universal

A soft, adjustable neck brace is used for many applications. It restricts movement and helps to hold the neck in place. It can be adjusted with the hook and loop fastener on the back of the brace. The pALS utilized this many times while in the manual wheelchair and during middle-stage ALS when transitioning from the cervical collar. It is soft, so more comfortable than the cervical collar, but extremely hot, especially in the summer months.

Neck Brace, Headmaster Collar™

The pALS was getting very hot trying to utilize other neck braces, so this one was appealing due to its structure containing less material than other neck braces. It is a tube design with cloth covering the tube. The chin rests on top of the tube on a chin pad, which is just an extra piece of material. Many things were tried to make this more comfortable for the pALS. We tried inserting gel into the chin pad portion and on the sides of the tube under the chin going toward the neck. The gel was one centimeter thick and cut from a motorcycle seat gel pad designed to aid in shock absorption. The Headmaster Collar was worn on many occasions but was extremely uncomfortable and really did not support the neck. It is definitely a neck brace that will either be liked or disliked by the pALS. There probably is no in-between. Also, it is somewhat pricey and likely not covered by insurance, so do some research on this one before purchasing. The pALS used the device in middle-stage ALS.

Neck Reading Light

This was received as a gift, after a family member witnessed the cALS using the light of a cell phone to illuminate inside the pALS' nose and ears. It is flexible and adjustable on the neck; however, it was only hung on the neck to better see when cutting finger and toenails. It worked well and was either held in the hand or hung on the lift recliner for use with the nose or ears.

Non-Invasive Ventilator

Despite having claustrophobia issues, the pALS agreed to try a non-invasive ventilator when his lung capacity was decreasing in late-stage ALS. All mask types were tried and at various pressures, but the pALS was still having difficulty. Finally, a "sip and puff" option was presented, where the pALS could just sip on a large plastic, straw-like structure with a mouthpiece, as needed, rather than having to wear a mask. The sip and puff was attached to the portable table and placed next to the lift recliner. This option worked really well for the pALS.

Note: The pALS could not sip through a regular straw, so there was concern that the "sip and puff" might not work. However, there was no issue with using it. The pALS really did not like having a breathing device, and it was not until end-stage ALS that he was willing to use it a little each day.

Non-Slip Pads

If the pALS has a lift recliner on a hard surface, some non-slip grips may be a good idea. We tried out several before we found a solution that worked moderately well. We started with vinyl cups and then went on to non-skid round gripper pads. Both worked okay, since the pALS was able to adjust in the lift recliner on his own. But the time came when the pALS needed to be pulled up more after initially sitting/being placed in the lift recliner, and those pads didn't hold the chair from moving on the floor. Some anti-slip furniture rail pads that were each 30 inches long were purchased. Although not perfect, they were able to grip the floor better than the round pads. These were used during middle- through end-stage ALS.

Non-Verbal Communication

There will likely come a time when the pALS is unable to communicate verbally. Whether it is by a shake of the head, use of the AAC, or it is just faster and easier to get an answer with some non-verbal communication, it is helpful to have a system in place before it is too late to establish one; for example, an eye-blinking system where the pALS blinks twice for yes and once for no. If the pALS still has slight movement of a thumb, that movement could denote an itch or alert that there is something going on in the lower body, etc. Maybe a smile with a tilt of the neck, while the neck can move, is a request for something that is used frequently. Whatever it may be, having something in place is helpful for all concerned.

Note: The non-verbal communication we utilized was established either on purpose, like the eye blinking, or perhaps because at one time the pALS was trying to express something and could not, so he made a gesture of some sort, like the slight movement of the thumb, which signified an itch, and the communication stuck. Many things are trial and error; however, being proactive and getting some signs in place early is beneficial. It can be used at any stage of ALS. Trying to choose gestures that may not have to be adjusted as the disease progresses is recommended; however, since everyone progresses differently, there may still have to be some adjustments made. The eye blinking proved beneficial for not only the cALS but also visitors, therapists, and medical professionals.

Oxygen Concentrator

The respiratory equipment company inadvertently delivered a home oxygen concentrator to the pALS during late-stage ALS, for one day. The pALS tried it and preferred it over the non-invasive ventilator, although the machines serve two different functions. The pALS qualified for a home oxygen concentrator two months later. It was worn for a good portion of the day and night for two weeks, during end-stage ALS, as the pALS felt he could breathe much more easily wearing it.

Phone/Phone Case

A heavy-duty phone case that will protect the cell phone if dropped, especially one with an opening at the bottom that can accommodate a wrist strap, is recommended. This is beneficial in early- and middle-stage ALS, when walking without assistance or walking with a rollator, for keeping the phone from falling out of reach in the lift chair, or just for ease of holding onto the strap rather than the phone.

Pill Crusher, Electric

RAUGEE™ Cordless electric pill crusher that quickly turns medications or vitamins into a dissolvable powder makes crushing, especially large pills, a lot faster and easier, and several can be processed at one time. The challenge is using a brush to empty the pill crusher to ensure all the powder makes it into the water to be dissolved, which is doable. This was used middle-stage and into the first part of late-stage ALS when there were larger pills that needed to be crushed.

Pill Crusher, Manual

This is a plastic container with a top and bottom designed to crush pills when the top is tightened. This was utilized daily from middle- through end-stage ALS.

Pill Cutter and Splitter

This plastic device, approximately 1 inch by 3 inches, has a blade that will easily split medications or vitamins in half or quarters. This was used during all stages of ALS.

Pill Organizer

It is helpful to have at least one pill organizer. We utilized a seven-day pill organizer that had compartments for morning and evening medications (am/pm). This was used for all stages of ALS. We also had a separate seven-day pill organizer for supplements. This one just had one large compartment for each day and was utilized from early- until middle-stage ALS, after which it came time to transition to liquid supplements.

Portable Ramp

A portable or possibly even permanent ramp may be needed at the pALS' place of residence, as well as at places that they may visit. Consider the elevation at all the residence doors. Is a small or even a large ramp needed? Which door(s) will be used most often? Can the ramp be moved from door to door as needed, rather than placing a ramp at every door? Since the door to the garage was the best choice for us as far as entering and exiting the house was concerned, a 24-inch-long by 28-inch-wide foldable aluminum ramp that could take up to 600 pounds in weight was purchased. This ramp was small and could be moved around easily, including to the back door so that the pALS could sit on the back patio as well. It was purchased during early-stage ALS to make it easier to navigate elevations and was used through end-stage ALS.

Think about social gatherings at friends' or family's houses. Are all places ADA accessible, or will a portable ramp be needed in order to get a wheelchair, walker or rollator inside? An 8-foot ramp with an 800-pound capacity was purchased in middle-stage ALS, that would accommodate any scenario for visits to other places. However, the ramp was somewhat pricey, and we only had the opportunity to use it once.

Pulse Oximeter

A portable fingertip pulse oximeter that could measure the oxygen level and pulse of the pALS was used throughout middle- and end-stage ALS.

Rollator Walker

A height-adjustable rollator walker with seat and backrest, 8-inch wheels, brakes and locking wheels was used. The rollator is lightweight and folds for easy transport. Some come with a storage pouch to hold personal belongings. The rollator was used for standing, long after the pALS lost the ability to walk. Amazingly, the pALS still had the upper body strength to hold himself up when his hands were placed on the rollator, despite having no use of his arms or hands. He continued standing until late-stage ALS, when the hip pain made it too difficult to do so. There are many different styles of walkers and rollator walkers available. This can sometimes be borrowed from an ALS organization, eliminating the need to purchase one.

Saline Nasal Mist

This item may be needed if the pALS uses oxygen or something that dries out the nose. This helps to provide some moisture in the nasal passages. It was used in late- and end-stage ALS.

Sinus Rinse

Originally done due to a minor procedure with the nose in middle-stage ALS, the sinus rinse used was by NeilMed® and was performed by the cALS using a manual squeeze bottle. The pALS did not enjoy the sinus rinse at first; however, once he had adjusted to it, he enjoyed having his nose feel clean. He would request a "nose douche" several times a week. Several months into middle-stage ALS, the pALS requested a pulsating nasal wash, so that he did not have to bend over a bowl, as that was getting difficult. Others with ALS had recommended the pulsating one since an individual can sit straight up to do it. But upon just showing the pALS the force of the stream of water coming out, he did not want to use the new pulsating one. The manual bottle was used as long as possible; however, before reaching late-stage ALS, the pALS could no longer bend over or blow his nose, so it could no longer be utilized.

Slick Sheet

This positioning bed pad, also known as a slick sheet, measures 48 inches by 40 inches. It was recommended by a physical therapist who thought the pad would make it easier to adjust the pALS in the lift recliner and possibly in bed too. Getting it underneath the pALS in the lift recliner was difficult, and the sheet was not helpful for us at all. It may be helpful for a pALS closer to average height, but not for one on the taller side.

Sling – Full Body, Mesh

A full-body mesh sling with an opening for the commode was tried with the Hoyer lift, in late-stage ALS, when attempting to get the pALS out of bed. The bottom portion raised before the top portion, so the pALS was leaning downward toward his head with his feet in the air. The sling was immediately lowered and was never used again.

Sling – Full Body, Solid Fabric

The Hoyer lift sling that is generally provided by the insurance company is a full-body sling that does not have any openings for the shower or commode. The only time this sling was utilized was initially when we were testing out the manual Hoyer lift. Nothing was wrong with the sling; it was just a preference, of liking the ease of use and comfort of the split leg sling.

Sling – Split Leg, Mesh

A full-body mesh divided leg sling with head and neck support for bathing and toileting was used with the Hoyer lift. We tried several slings, and this was the only sling that the pALS liked and used every day. It was the easiest to utilize in all applications, whether in bed, lift recliner, shower chair, spa/hot tub, toileting or wheelchair. In end-stage ALS, the pALS had lost a substantial amount of weight and reported that the split leg hurt his legs as it was cutting into the skin. Small towels were placed on the legs to block the sling from sinking into the skin too much, and they did just that. However, the pALS opted not to have any additional padding and to just use the sling as we always had. This was used during middle- through end-stage ALS.

Slip-in Sneakers

Slip-in sneakers allowed the pALS to put on his own shoes until late in middle-stage ALS and then allowed the cALS to easily put on/take off his shoes. There were two different types tried, both of the brand Skechers®. Only one of the styles worked well for the pALS, both in putting the shoes on as well as enabling him to stand due to a higher heel, until late-stage ALS. Those were the *Skechers Ultra Flex 3.0 – Right Away* model. The shoes were worn during middle- through end-stage ALS.

Stool Softener

Under the direction of a medical professional, there will likely be a time when the pALS will need a stool softener. There are many available; we chose MiraLAX®, since it was dissolvable and could be put through the pALS' feeding tube.

Suction Machine, Portable

This is another item where I cannot emphasize enough the need to be proactive in getting it early. We had one on standby about 10 months before it was needed. When the saliva starts flowing and cannot be swallowed, constant suctioning is required. Without this, the pALS will choke a lot and have saliva dribbling from the mouth. Different wands can be used with the machine; find one that is most comfortable for the pALS. The thinner ones tend to be more comfortable; however, our experience was that the pALS would lose control of the jaw, and when the teeth clamped down hard, the end of the wand was bitten off the thinner wands. In late- and end-stage ALS, a pediatric suction wand was utilized in the nose to assist with nasal secretions. The wands are interchangeable on the suction machine.

Transfer Disc

This device was recommended by the occupational therapist (OT) during middle-stage ALS. At this point, the pALS was no longer walking, but could use his rollator to pivot between equipment, such as from the wheelchair to the shower chair or from the lift recliner to the wheelchair. The transfer disc rotates 360 degrees to assist in turning the pALS. The OT attempted to demonstrate getting into the shower from the wheelchair, but had a hard time rotating the pALS. The pALS and cALS tried it from the toilet to the wheelchair and from the wheelchair to the lift recliner. It was difficult, but doable. The pALS, always searching for a better way, tried to rotate on one leg on the disc with his rollator. It was a good idea but did not quite work as he had hoped. We discontinued use of the transfer disc after trying to utilize it several times in one day.

Transfer Nursing Sling

This sling is 50 inches long and 9 inches wide with padded handles on each end. The inside is made of suede, and the outside of a durable Oxford material. It wraps more around the torso and is supposed to assist in getting the pALS up and/or for transferring the pALS.

Note: This sling was attempted on several occasions when the pALS was still semi-mobile, including attempts to loop it under the pALS to move him up in bed. In bed is the only time it somewhat worked. It never proved successful in lifting the pALS for a transfer.

Underwear

There are different types of fly openings for men that may assist when using the urinal. There is adaptive underwear for women as well. We experimented with a different fly opening for two days and one night in middle-stage ALS; however, the pALS was partial to a certain material, style and type of underwear, so no changes were made in this area.

Wheelchair, Electric

An electric wheelchair is something that should be explored as early as possible. This is a very costly item and there may be other ways of obtaining one than purchasing, such as borrowing one from an ALS organization. The drawback of a borrowed wheelchair is that it is not made specifically for the pALS and may not be the right size and could lack accessories and comfort.

If purchasing, carefully consider all available options and try to imagine what the future will look like for the pALS. As with everything, the costs increase with each additional item, and insurance may only cover certain types of accessories—such as a specific type of seat. Get what you can up front, because as the disease progresses, there may be something that is needed, and when the time comes, you will not have it. Things can always be added down the line; however, as previously discussed, requesting things through doctors, therapists, insurance and vendors tends to take considerable time.

The pALS ordered two items for his wheelchair that were extremely beneficial:

- Seat elevator – used to raise the chair to a higher elevation for sitting at a bar/island or for exiting the chair. This is something which *Team Gleason* assisted with financially.

- Rear attendant controls – a joystick and speed control to drive the chair. Also, a set of buttons in the rear to control the tilt, rising and lowering of the seat and foot plates.

Other things to take into consideration:

- Ability Drive – An alternative to a joystick, where the user drives with the eyes, utilizing a program on an eye-gaze device. The pALS tested this method in late-stage ALS. The technician reported that the pALS was able to use it much better than most on the first attempt. However, based on the slow responsiveness and low ability to use it outdoors, the pALS determined that it was not a good fit. In addition, it required an older AAC than the pALS had, so a different eye-gaze device would have to be utilized for the wheelchair and that would not provide the pALS with all the outside communication, such as text messaging, while in the wheelchair. This aspect needs to be taken into consideration before deciding on an AAC device too.

- Joystick – the standard compact joystick may be difficult to work with, depending on the pALS' hand function. There are other options available, and this is something that may be switched more than once until one can find the perfect option. The one that worked best in our situation was a U-shaped handle that had a waterfall edge and wings on each side so the hand would not slip off. While the pALS' hand had to be placed on this joystick just perfectly, it worked well while he had the function of his hand. Unfortunately, about five months after getting the wheelchair, the pALS was unable to drive and had to rely on the cALS.

- Armrests – for added comfort and support, consider a gel-type armrest rather than the standard armrest.

- Headrest – It is strongly recommended to think this through thoroughly before deciding on the type. The headrest that was recommended for the pALS' chair was not a good fit for someone who lacked head control and could not keep his head from falling forward. There was a strap with a circumference of a small shoestring on a pulley system, going through a piece of leather, that went around the forehead and was supposed to hold it in place. Besides the extreme discomfort, it did not work either. A new headrest was ordered and received almost six months after the initial conversation about the headrest began. Meanwhile, the pALS could not use his wheelchair unless absolutely needed, as there was no way to hold his head in place…except for the head controls, which assisted slightly.

- Head Controls – These turn the wheelchair off and on and change the function, so that the pALS can adjust the seat, turn on lights, etc. They were beneficial at first, except when in a vehicle, as the bouncing makes the head hit them, and as a result, the wheelchair turns off and on constantly. Also, as head control declined, the controls couldn't be used and had to be disconnected, as the pALS' head would just lie on them. Depending on the headrest that is selected, head controls may not be an option.

- Supports – Thigh and trunk supports were never utilized. Towards end-stage ALS, the thigh supports would have been beneficial; however, due to the overhang of the seat, the supports could not be inserted into the track of the chair.

- Seat – There is a standard seat that insurance covers, although the pALS reported it being very hard and uncomfortable. A ROHO™ had been purchased for the lift recliner and was being utilized in the wheelchair as well, while trying to obtain one through insurance. Several months down the line, a *CG Air Cushion* was gifted to the pALS that proved to be more comfortable than the one he was trying to obtain through insurance. Although it was not exactly the size needed, it became the seat that was used in the wheelchair and lift recliner.

Wheelchair or Transport Chair, Manual

Walking may become tiring in the early stages of ALS, and even a short distance can be hard. Going to appointments becomes burdensome for the pALS because it is usually quite a hike to get inside. Perhaps the pALS just wants to enjoy a walk or some fresh air without getting too worn out. Having a lightweight wheelchair or transport chair is quite helpful and allows for all these things to be accomplished. The one the pALS utilized had swing-away footrests, arms that flipped up, an 18-inch seat and folded for transport. This was utilized from early- until middle-stage ALS, when an electric loaner wheelchair arrived, pending delivery of the pALS' permanent electric wheelchair.

Chapter 6

Eating and Drinking

EATING AND DRINKING were maintained for as long as possible. Despite still being able to do both, the pALS opted to be proactive and get a feeding tube about six months before it was needed full-time. However, this is a personal choice, and this guidebook does not promote doing anything one way or another. If a feeding tube is being explored, consider being proactive and getting it early. In our case, it proved to be beneficial. Since it was inserted early, there was no scrambling when the need for it arose. The transition from being able to eat and drink by mouth to being unable to do so happened literally between breakfast and lunch. Prior to using it full-time, it was used for medications and hydration. As it became harder for the pALS to eat, mostly due to tiredness of the jaw, either lunch or a snack would be supplemented with liquid nutrition. This would give the jaw a rest and ensure that the pALS was consuming enough calories.

Despite being unable to feed himself, the pALS still enjoyed having meals with others while he was able to eat orally. We would eat each meal together and use the "one for you, one for me" method, where each person would take a bite by turns. After switching full-time to the feeding tube, the cALS would still sit next to him and eat, until such time as the saliva got so bad it seemed that the sight and smell of food was increasing saliva production. The pALS insisted it was not; however, the cALS still chose to eat away from him.

Below are some items we tried, with varying results.

Adaptive Silverware

Gripping things was becoming difficult for the pALS, so cooking and holding silverware properly was becoming a challenge. The silverware could be manipulated if held more like a child would hold it, gripping the handle like a fist with all fingers wrapped around. This technique worked for about six months after diagnosis, before beginning to use adaptive utensils. Adaptive utensils are made for those who have a weak grip. Some come with just larger handles and others have larger handles with curved heads. The pALS found the ones with larger handles and curved heads the easiest to use.

Adult Bib

A vinyl adult bib that is large in size, 34 inches long by 18 inches wide, and covers the entire torso, is useful. The one we used was waterproof and washable and snapped around the back of the neck. The bottom also had a fold to catch any spilled food. It even had the phrase, "I freaking spill everything" printed on it, to add a little humor. The bib was still utilized when the pALS could no longer feed himself, but since he was generally fed in the lift recliner, the bib was just placed over him and not snapped around the neck. It was also easily washable by applying some dish soap to the front and using a non-scratch all-purpose cleaning pad.

Baby Fresh Food Feeder

A teething feeder made of Nitrosamine enabled the pALS to chew on the mesh and taste the juice of the fruit inside. This was first introduced in late-stage ALS, about seven months after the last time the pALS could orally take food and drink. We tried it because the pALS was missing drinking liquids orally so much. It was preferred over the baby push pop feeder, but could only be used on two occasions. It would be beneficial to attempt at an earlier stage of ALS.

Baby Push Pop Feeder

A silicone fruit feeder for fresh and frozen fruit allowed for some flavor in the mouth when the pALS could no longer eat or drink orally. This was first introduced in late-stage ALS, about seven months after the last time the pALS could orally take food and drink. It was used once and worked okay; however, the fresh food feeder was preferred. It would be beneficial to attempt at an earlier stage of ALS.

Bag Feeding

Literally overnight, the pALS went from eating the recommended daily amount to barely being able to eat without feeling full. The dietician recommended bag feeding, rather than bolus feeding, to slow the process. The pALS tried this for a short time and did not like it for food, but didn't mind it as much for water and hydration. Within three weeks, we went back to bolus feeding since it was the method preferred by the pALS.

Blender

A blender was used to blend fruit, vegetables or both together for smoothies. The pALS drank smoothies through a straw in early- and parts of middle-stage ALS. Adding water to the smoothie not only helps it blend but also makes it thinner and easier to drink while also providing hydration for the pALS. When the pALS could no longer drink through a straw in middle-stage ALS, the smoothie was made thicker so that it could be spoon-fed to the pALS. Whey protein and collagen were also added to the smoothies, especially as the pALS' ability to eat food was reducing.

The blender can also be used to chop or puree food as the pALS' ability to eat lessens. We also used it for chopping dry oatmeal to make it finer and easier to swallow. The pALS did not mind having food chopped a little finer in the blender; however, he was not a big fan of having foods blended together and pureed.

BOOST™ Very High Calorie

Nutritional drinks with higher calories (530) and protein (22g) than the average BOOST were used to supplement the diet when chewing was getting harder. BOOST, or the nutritional drink of choice, is something that one may be able to find through the *Oley Foundation* so that it does not have to be purchased out-of-pocket.

Catheter Tip Syringe

When the pALS got his feeding tube, we began purchasing 60 mL (milliliter) sterile plastic catheter tip syringes in packs of 10 to flush the tube. After transitioning to liquid nutrition, we continued to buy these syringes, because they were larger, of better quality, and operated more smoothly than those supplied by the nutrition company. The larger size made it easier to keep the pALS hydrated and to flush the tube before and after feeding or administering medications.

For bolus feeding, a syringe with the plunger removed was used to make measuring approximately two ounces of nutrition easier. This was especially helpful when the pALS could not eat as much at one time or needed just two to four ounces of nutrition before bedtime, as the liquid food could be poured directly from the container into the syringe.

A 10 mL syringe was tried during middle-stage ALS for medications but was not found suitable by the cALS. Toward the end of late- and end-stage ALS, the pALS was taking more liquid medications than before and it was much easier to just utilize multiple 10 mL syringes—many of which came with the medications—than to use a different syringe or container.

Chopping Finely

As it was getting harder to swallow and not choke on food, chopping things very finely helped. The pALS still wanted to eat chicken and ground turkey. The chicken was chopped almost hair fine and the ground turkey cooked very finely, constantly moving it in the pan so as to not leave any big chunks. Pureeing meat in a blender was not something the pALS fancied in our case; however, it could be an option in other cases.

Collagen Peptides

Hydrolyzed Type 1 and Type 3 collagen peptides were utilized, hoping they might benefit the pALS. The unflavored collagen was generally added and blended into a smoothie in early- and middle-stage ALS. In late- and end-stage ALS, it was added to water and administered through the feeding tube.

Note: This section is for information only and is not intended to prescribe or promote any supplement(s) for other pALS.

Double Handled Sippy Cup (Cold Beverages)

This is a plastic cup for adults with limited mobility, having one handle on each side. The lid has a spout that protrudes out of the top as well as a lid that allows for a straw. It is touted as spillproof, but a limited amount of the liquid can escape. It is lightweight and easy to lift and drink, even with assistance if needed. This cup was utilized until approximately two months before the pALS could no longer drink liquids with the assistance of the cALS.

Double Handled Sippy Cup (Hot Beverages)

This plastic cup for adults has one handle on each side and a weighted bottom so it will not tip. It could be used for cold beverages as well; it just isn't as easy to lift for the pALS as the disease progresses, due to the weight. The lid has a spout that protrudes out of the top. A limited amount of liquid can escape. This was easy for the pALS to use for coffee in the earlier stages. When the pALS was no longer able to lift it, it was used with the assistance of the cALS, until the pALS could no longer drink liquids orally.

Easier to Swallow Foods

Finding foods that are easier to swallow and do not require a lot of chewing is beneficial, especially as the disease progresses. The jaw gets tired from chewing, and the pALS loses the ability to finish a meal. Some foods that were utilized a lot were different flavors of applesauce and yogurt, stovetop and instant pudding, mashed potatoes, poached eggs, cream of wheat with added honey and cinnamon, and oatmeal (first blending the dry oats before cooking to make the oats smaller). Cutting wild blueberries in half or quarters, depending on the size, to add to the oatmeal and cream of wheat, would add some variety of flavor in addition to the honey. On rare occasions, brown sugar was added to the oatmeal to switch up the flavor a bit. Applesauce and yogurt were used to take medications when the pALS could no longer drink water orally. Also, small shell pasta with a lot of sauce, refried beans and macaroni and cheese were some other options. The macaroni and cheese with the creamy, liquid cheese was used to provide more moisture. The finely chopped meat discussed earlier was also an option, with a lot of dipping sauce to enable the meat to be swallowed. Everything needed a lot of sauce to help it go down.

Extension Tubes

The pALS had a low-profile *MIC-KEY* button-type feeding tube. For both bolus and bag feeding, a 12-inch extension tube with a catheter tip was used. It locked securely in place to prevent leakage and had a clamp that could be opened or closed to allow/not allow liquid through. The only difference with bag feeding was that a plastic cone had to be attached to the end of the tube on the bag and inserted into the end of the extension tube to secure it.

For medications, a 12-inch tube with a clamp was also used; however, the tube was narrower and had an ENFit® connector, rather than a catheter connector. It also had a "Y" port at the end, with ports of different sizes: one designed to accommodate a larger syringe, such as a 60 mL syringe, and the other for a smaller syringe, such as a 10 mL one. The larger port was used for flushing with water, and the smaller port was used for administering medications. This tube was used more during late- and end-stage ALS, whereas the other tube was generally utilized earlier in disease progression.

Note: All feeding tube products were washed at least once daily with soap and hot water and then always rinsed after each use. They were washed individually, never soaked in water. If something needed to be scrubbed, such as the container or syringe used for medication, food, etc., a clean paper towel was used, and never a sponge or anything that might contain bacteria. When running the dishwasher, all feeding tube "equipment" was placed in the dishwasher to ensure it was thoroughly washed. If the plunger of a syringe becomes hard to move after washing, a small amount of cooking oil can be applied to the rubber stopper to lubricate it. Be careful not to use anything toxic to lubricate the plunger, as it is being used to administer food and water to a living person.

Fast Hydration Electrolyte Solution

The fast hydration electrolyte solution has double the electrolytes, compared to other electrolyte options, to assist with hydrating the pALS quickly. Due to the amount of saliva, the pALS liked to limit water intake as much as possible in late- and end-stage ALS and instead opted to utilize electrolytes as needed.

Ice Cube Trays

When the pALS was unable to drink orally, different beverages, such as lemonade, were frozen in ice trays. The cubes were then crushed into small ice shards and placed in the pALS' mouth to moisten it and provide a bit of sensory pleasure.

Large Latex Straws

Early on, large latex straws were purchased for ease of drinking water and smoothies. The straws worked well in both stainless steel and plastic tumblers, although the plastic tumblers were easiest for the pALS to hold and grip.

Liquid Thickener

There are many brands of food and beverage thickeners available, although the pALS did not try this until late-stage ALS, just weeks before end-stage ALS. The pALS missed drinking water so much that we were trying anything for him to be able to drink water and taste other beverages. The brand purchased was Thick It®. It is flavorless and does thicken beverages but takes some experimentation to get the right thickness. We first tried it in a one-ounce plastic disposable portion cup and later in a sippy cup. We also tried spoon feeding the liquid to the pALS—anything for him to get a little taste. Obviously, making the beverage thicker made it seem less like drinking a liquid.

Oral Care Swabs

Disposable sponges on a stick were used to moisten the mouth. We used these not only with plain water but also with beverages that the pALS liked, so that he could taste something different. Occasionally, mouthwash was also added to the sponge to sanitize the pALS' teeth and tongue.

Note: The sponges were used much more in end-stage ALS to remove dry saliva from the cheeks and tongue. To do this, the sponges were used dry.

Protein, Whey

This was unflavored and used in smoothies and water to add additional protein into the pALS' diet, especially when he was not able to get enough through food as eating diminished.

Supplements

When the pALS could swallow, he would take several supplements orally, including Omega-3, B12, D3, K2, magnesium and a probiotic powder containing prebiotics. When swallowing became difficult, the supplements were used in a liquid form that could be put down the feeding tube, with the exception of the magnesium and probiotics, which were dissolved in water. The probiotic was also added to a smoothie, rather than dissolved, when possible. A multivitamin was added to the routine when transitioning to liquids.

Note: Ensure that anything being put down the feeding tube will not clog or disintegrate the tube. Flush with plenty of water to ensure that all residues are removed.

Tumblers, Plastic

Stackable plastic water tumblers, 20 ounces each, were used for smoothies. The tumblers easily accommodated the large latex straws, and they made it fairly easy for the pALS to drink most of the contents from the tumbler. These would have been beneficial during early-stage ALS, but were not purchased until the beginning of middle-stage ALS. For a short time after purchase, into the early part of middle-stage ALS, the pALS was able to hold the tumblers.

TummyDrops®

Lozenges containing ginger that may help an upset stomach. For a short time, the pALS tried these drops to assist when he was having issues with his stomach, when first diagnosed with ALS.

The following outlines the ALS stage(s) in which each item was utilized.

Early-Stage ALS

The pALS could still eat most foods; however, chewing and swallowing started becoming more difficult within eight months after diagnosis.

- Adaptive silverware
- Adult bib

- Blender for smoothies
- Collagen
- Double-handled sippy cup (hot and cold beverages)
- Large latex straws
- Protein, Whey
- Supplements
- TummyDrops

Middle-Stage ALS

From nine to 14 months after diagnosis, eating became extremely difficult, and the pALS' jaw would get tired. The pALS could also no longer use silverware or adaptive silverware and could only use his hands to eat through month nine. After that, he needed assistance eating. At about month eleven, one meal and/or snack per day was supplemented with liquid nutrition to alleviate some of the fatigue, and softer or finely chopped foods were introduced. Just after the fifteenth month, the pALS could no longer eat or drink.

- Adult bib
- BOOST and other liquid nutrition recommended by the dietitian
- Blender for smoothies
- Catheter-tip syringe
- Chopping finely
- Collagen peptides
- Double-handled sippy cup (hot and cold beverages) with assistance
- Easier-to-swallow foods
- Extension tubes
- Ice cube trays
- Large latex straws
- Protein, Whey
- Supplements
- Tumblers, Plastic

Late-Stage ALS

The pALS didn't mind not being able to eat so much; however, he really missed drinking liquids, especially water. We were experimenting with different things to try and satisfy the beverage craving. The pALS wanted to stop taking supplements toward the end of late-stage ALS, so they were used intermittently as requested.

- Baby fresh-food feeder (used twice)
- Baby push-pop feeder (used once)
- Bag feeding (used intermittently up to three weeks)
- Catheter-tip syringe
- Collagen peptides
- Disposable portion cups
- Double-handled sippy cup (hot beverages) – for ease of use
- Extension tubes
- Fast hydration electrolyte solution
- Liquid thickener
- Oral care swabs
- Protein, whey
- Supplements (as requested)

End-Stage ALS

The pALS was not interested in continuing to take supplements at this point. However, he thought that he noticed a difference in his hip pain when taking magnesium versus not, so he opted to add that supplement back into his daily routine.

- Catheter-tip syringe
- Collagen peptides
- Extension tubes
- Fast-hydration electrolyte solution
- Oral care swabs
- Protein, Whey
- Supplements (as requested)

Chapter 7

Oral Care

ORAL CARE IS important to keep the teeth and mouth feeling fresh and to minimize germs and prevent their spread throughout the body. Part of the morning and evening routines included toothbrushing. When the pALS was still eating orally, teeth would be brushed before and after eating in the morning or throughout the day as needed, and then before going to bed at night. When the pALS was still mobile, toothbrushing was done standing over the sink in the bathroom. As mobility declined, it was done either in the wheelchair or the lift recliner. Towards the end of being able to swallow pills by mouth, the pills were being swallowed with applesauce or dairy-free yogurt instead of water. When that was done and a few pills were required to be taken after getting into bed at night, the toothbrushing would take place with the pALS sitting up in the adjustable bed. Eventually, when no food or pills were being taken orally, we returned to just brushing in the lift recliner.

Dental Floss

A standard, waxed dental floss was found to be easiest and fastest to use. This was used in early- and middle-stage ALS. As the disease progressed, it was harder to floss anything other than the front teeth due to jaw fatigue and jaw clamping.

Disposable Portion Cups

One-ounce plastic disposable portion cups were used from middle- to end-stage ALS, enabling the pALS to utilize mouthwash. These were also used when attempting to sample some beverages in late-stage ALS.

Emesis Basin

A kidney-shaped basin was utilized when brushing teeth in the lift recliner or bed, once standing over the sink became difficult. The basin catches toothpaste, mouthwash, etc. and is washable and reusable. It was used from middle- to end-stage ALS.

Mobile Dentist

The pALS wanted badly to have professional teeth cleaning in middle- and late-stage ALS; however, there were no mobile dentists available in the area. We improvised by purchasing a professional tartar scraper tool, but this was not ideal. Letting a professional do the job is much better and recommended. There are many locations where mobile dentists are available; just check the area where you live.

Mouthwash

Mouthwash was used as a mouth rinse after brushing, throughout middle-stage ALS. In late- and end-stage ALS, the pALS could not tolerate toothpaste, so it was used to brush teeth as well as rinse the mouth. As saliva worsened, mouthwash was used several times throughout the day, as needed, to help remove bacteria, and hopefully reduce saliva. Despite experimenting with various brands and products, Crest Pro Health™ remained the pALS' preferred mouthwash.

Toothbrush, Adult

A soft, manual adult toothbrush was used during early-stage ALS until transitioning to an electric toothbrush. A tongue scraper on the back of an adult toothbrush was utilized through end-stage ALS.

Toothbrush, Youth

A soft, manual youth toothbrush was used from middle- through end-stage ALS. The small head of the toothbrush is easier to move around and get to the hard-to-reach areas, especially as the disease progresses.

Toothbrush, Electric

The pALS utilized an electric toothbrush from early-stage ALS until middle-stage ALS. The one that was used was recognized as Americans with Disabilities Act (ADA) compliant.

Xlear® with Xylitol

These are sinus rinse packets and were used in late-stage ALS for assistance in drying up saliva. The rinse was applied using an oral sponge to swab it around the mouth. The pALS reported that this worked better than any prescription medication tried; however, he did not like the way it dried saliva in his mouth, as the dry saliva would get stuck on his cheeks, teeth, and tongue.

Chapter 8

Bathing

THE PALS WAS accustomed to taking showers frequently every day prior to diagnosis. When the time came that assistance was needed with showering, he got a shower every night. As the disease progressed, showers were taken earlier in the day, accounting for the resulting fatigue. In late-stage ALS, shower times were determined by the amount of saliva being produced at a given time. We headed to the shower when there was less saliva, which was generally shortly after getting out of bed. As he got closer to end-stage ALS, showering frequency reduced to every other day. During end-stage ALS, it often was every two to three days. In between, he was wiped down with a warm washcloth and his favorite soap.

As showering became more exhausting for the pALS, we tried to accomplish as much as possible before getting out of the lift recliner, such as cleaning the face, ears and neck. This made showering faster and reduced the amount of time that the head would have to hang forward in the shower.

When a solid seat was installed on the shower chair, his bottom could no longer be washed inside the shower since there was no seat opening. Once up in the Hoyer lift, his bottom and the backs of his legs touching the seat would be washed with warm water and soap, using two washcloths (one for soap and one for rinsing). Then he would be placed on the shower chair and taken to the shower where the rest of his body would be washed. After the shower, his hair and body were towel dried, and the drying was completed with a hairdryer, as described below.

Aftershave Lotion

Face lotion applied after a shave and shower assisted in moisturizing skin and mitigated any irritation from shaving.

Aquaphor®

This jelly was used occasionally, especially when first getting the feeding tube inserted, to relieve itching and irritation on the skin around the tube. The irritation was mostly caused by the tape used to hold the gauze in place. In end-stage ALS, the area around the tube began to itch again, and the jelly was applied as needed to the skin around the feeding tube after showering.

Baby Powder

The powder was utilized throughout all stages of ALS for leg creases that might sweat and cause odor and irritation from sitting. It was also used in lieu of deodorant in the latter part of early-stage ALS into middle-stage ALS when the pALS had been showering himself and the armpits were irritated from being unable to remove deodorant. Once the armpits were healed, the use of deodorant was resumed.

Body Wipes/Sponges

Several different types of body wipes and sponges were tried, to see if they would be a good alternative to showering every day. They worked okay, but didn't give the same fresh feeling as showering or even using a washcloth with soap and water. The wipes are better than nothing, yet not ideal. They were tried in middle-stage ALS and a few times in end-stage ALS after getting out of the spa.

Bowl

A large plastic bowl was initially used for water to clean the feeding tube during the first six weeks after it was inserted. It was later used as a catcher when doing a nose douche or for hot water when doing a quick wipe down of the body or while washing the hands.

Cotton Swabs

These were utilized throughout all stages of ALS for the ears. They were also used to clean around the feeding tube once it was put in place and to clean inside the nose, "fishing", during middle- through end-stage ALS.

Deodorant

A combined antiperspirant and deodorant were used on the armpits. It was applied before dressing the pALS in the morning and after showering.

Dressing

When utilizing both the stationary and sliding shower chairs, the pALS was dressed in the bathroom, as he could still use his rollator for balance. When we began using the Nuprodx Mobility® shower chair, once the pALS had been dried with the hairdryer, deodorant was added to the armpits. The shower chair was then moved from a reclined to an upright position, and the pALS pulled forward so his back could be dried as well. Afterward, his shirt was put on, and the Hoyer lift sling was tucked behind his back. The shower chair was reclined again, and the sling wrapped around his legs so he could be lifted by the Hoyer lift to complete the drying process. Once dry, foot spray was applied before he was taken to his lift recliner to finish dressing.

Note: Initially, the shirt was not put on until the pALS was in the lift recliner; however, it was found beneficial to put it on after drying his back in the shower chair. This kept him warmer in the winter and prevented the sling from touching as much skin, reducing itching and scratching sensations—making him more comfortable all around.

Exfoliating Bath Gloves

As bathing became more tiring for the pALS in middle-stage ALS, we tried exfoliating gloves in hopes of speeding up the showering process by reducing fumbling with the loofah. However, just one minute into the shower, the pALS requested the gloves be removed and wanted to go back to the loofah.

Exfoliating Sponges

Single-use, square facial exfoliating sponges were used to clean the face. These were used during middle- through end-stage ALS. The pALS preferred them over using just a washcloth or a facial wipe.

Facial Soap

Cleansing soap was used specifically for the face, with the exfoliating sponges, during middle- through end-stage ALS.

Facial Wipe

Cleansing wipes were used specifically for the face. Tried in middle-stage ALS for a short time, the pALS did not like the way the wipes made his face feel. However, there are many different wipes on the market, so this method may have worked with a different type or brand of wipe.

Foot Spray

Foot powder spray was utilized during middle- through end-stage ALS after the pALS got out of the shower. It helped him feel fresher after showering and before putting on socks and shoes.

Grab Bars

Hard plastic grab bars with suction cups assisted with balance. The grab bars come in a set of two and were placed on the tile shower to assist the pALS in getting up, from the stationary shower chair, as well as giving the pALS something to hold onto by the edge of the shower while being dried. The grab bars were very secure on the tile, as long as they were not placed on a grout line, and the suction cups allowed them to be relocated as needed. These were used during early- through the early part of middle-stage ALS. Once the sliding shower chair was introduced, the plastic grab bars were removed from the shower, as they were no longer needed.

Emesis Basin

A kidney-shaped basin was utilized for oral care and cleaning around and under the feeding tube after showering. It is advisable to wash the basin with soap and hot water after each use and to have multiple basins so those used for oral care are not also used for bathing. These were used during middle- through end-stage ALS.

Hairdryer

Used not only for hair, the dryer was initially used for parts of the body that could be prone to chafing if left damp, such as armpits, hands and feet. It was also used as a precaution to ensure hands were completely dry before grabbing the rollator, when that was being used, and feet were dry before putting on shoes and socks. As the disease progressed and the pALS became less mobile, after towel drying, the entire body—except for the arms and legs —was dried using a hairdryer. Some of it was done in the shower chair, including the hair, neck, chest, hands, armpits, feet and back, while the rest was completed in the Hoyer lift.

Loofah

A loofah mesh bath sponge was utilized throughout all stages of ALS, except for a short time in the early and middle stages when the pALS was still trying to shower himself. During that time, silicone scrubbers were used.

Lotion

Moisturizing body lotion kept the pALS' skin moist, and was applied as needed.

Oatmeal Soap

Colloidal oatmeal soap was used to clean around and under the feeding tube. It is a gentle soap that is fragrance and chemical free, so it did not cause any irritation. The feeding tube was cleaned daily after showering. If a shower was skipped, the feeding tube would still be cleaned.

Shower/Bathmat

A 35-inch by 16-inch non-skid mat was used for the shower. The mat had suction cups that kept it secure and holes that allowed drainage. This is something that can be utilized from early- through end-stage ALS, providing the shower chair is stationary. It provides the extra grip needed to keep the pALS' feet from slipping when leg and foot control begins to decline. If utilizing a rolling shower chair that needs to roll over the area where the mat is placed, consider removing the mat.

Shower Arm Diverter

If purchasing a handheld shower head, be aware that you will likely need to purchase a shower arm diverter as well, to keep the original shower head in place. The diverter will allow the handheld shower head to be attached and will allow either the original shower head or the handheld shower head to be utilized independently.

Shower Cap

This may be needed for the pALS or the cALS throughout all stages of ALS. In our case, it was used by the cALS from middle- to end-stage ALS to help with overspray.

Shower Chair, MacGyver

Not wanting to be wiped down only outside the shower, the pALS developed a workaround to ensure daily showers continued when it seemed the days of getting him into the shower with the current equipment were numbered. The Nuprodx shower chair arrived in time, so this method was not attempted; however, it is worth mentioning in case it may be helpful to others.

The supplies/accessories needed are:

- Two shower hoses
- Shower hose extension adapter
- Handheld shower head with on/off switch
- Plastic children's pool
- Loofah / soap / shampoo
- Hoyer lift
- Split leg mesh sling
- Pump (optional)

Connect the hoses and put the handheld shower on the end. Place the children's pool outside the shower and dangle the pALS over the pool in the Hoyer lift. Use the handheld shower head, loofah, soap and shampoo to wash and rinse the pALS. Empty the pool water into the shower, or invest in a pump and empty water into the shower that way.

Shower Chair/Commode Chair, Nuprodx

The pALS loved daily showers and had reached a point where transferring him from the wheelchair and rollator to the sliding shower chair was becoming too dangerous. The *Nuprodx* MC6000RSTilt is a shower/commode chair we had been looking at but could not afford. We had already gotten assistance from Team Gleason for the electric wheelchair seat elevator and did not want to request additional help for this purchase. This chair was appealing due to its design having a bridge system, so that the shower chair could go over the raised ledge, which would normally require stepping over to get into the shower. We were quite fortunate and had a fully equipped chair, large enough for the pALS, donated to us by someone who no longer needed it.

It was used solely as a shower chair but had a cut-out seat for the commode. When the pALS began losing weight and growing weaker, the seat was becoming uncomfortable if he was not positioned squarely on the seat when placed by the Hoyer lift. A solid seat was purchased through the manufacturer of the shower chair, to resolve the issue.

The shower chair separates from the bridge and can be rolled around in the shower. The handheld shower unit was placed at a height that was compatible with the shower chair, so that the chair could be rolled up to it and it would be as if the pALS was actually standing in a shower with the water flowing down his neck and back. He would close his eyes and let the water flow down, saying that for those 10 minutes, he felt "normal". This device was received in middle-stage and used through end-stage ALS.

Shower Chair/Commode Chair, Reclining

This reclining and adjustable multi-function shower chair with adjustable headrest, arm rests, footrests and commode was purchased online and was very costly. It was a horrible chair. It, in fact, would not recline, and the seat was so hard and uncomfortable that the pALS could not tolerate sitting on it. It was attempted as a commode chair on two occasions but never as a shower chair. We discontinued use of it and went back to using the sliding shower chair for a couple more weeks. This was attempted in middle-stage ALS.

Shower Chair, Sliding

This sliding shower chair with a transfer bench had a swivel seat equipped with thick padding, armrests that flip up, a seatback and adjustable legs. There was a short ledge on the shower, and the two outside legs of the sliding shower chair were placed on the outside of the shower ledge to enable the pALS to transfer more easily from/to the rollator. Once the pALS was seated, the seat was turned and pushed inside the shower to the opposite side, where it locked in place. The shower curtain was split about 24 inches up in two places to fit around the legs that were outside the shower. Due to the rapid progression of the disease, we got about five months of use out of this shower chair. If purchasing a shower chair, it would be beneficial to start with this one rather than a stationary chair, which will require upgrading at some point anyway.

Shower Chair, Stationary

This is an adjustable-height shower chair with a backrest and armrest. The seat is flat and in three segmented sections, with dimensions of 12 inches deep by 19 inches wide. It was utilized during early-stage and slightly into middle-stage ALS.

Shower Curtain

The shower had about a 36-inch opening with no glass. This allowed for a lot of cold air to hit the pALS, who was sitting in a shower chair that did not have a continuous stream of water overhead. The shower curtain allowed for the opening to be covered so that the cold air was not hitting the pALS. This was helpful all the time and especially during the winter months.

The shower curtain was still utilized when transitioning to the *Nuprodx* chair, which could be pushed to the opposite end of the shower to assist in keeping the cold air out. The challenge encountered with this in the latter part of late- and end-stage ALS was the difficulty breathing if steam built up inside the shower.

Shower Head Extension Hose

This flexible stainless-steel hose comes in varying lengths. A shower hose extension adapter can be used to connect two hoses if a longer hose is needed.

Shower Head Handheld with On/Off Switch

A high-pressure handheld shower head with an on/off switch is useful so that the water may be turned off if desired. Some come with a water flow that has more than one setting. The one we used had five settings; however, we tended to always use the same setting.

Note: Originally, a shower head with eight settings was purchased, but it had no on/off switch. We utilized this shower head for several months prior to purchasing the one with the on/off switch to replace it, which was a better fit for us.

Shower Head Holder

A suction shower head holder is required to hold the handheld shower head. The suction is a vacuum suction so that the holder can be relocated as needed. When we got the *Nuprodx* bath chair, the holder was moved up higher so that the water could hit the pALS on the back of the neck. This not only kept the pALS warmer but also better simulated a "real shower".

Shower Hose Extension Adapter

Made of solid stainless steel, this device can be used to connect two shower hoses together, to make it easier to rinse the pALS with a handheld shower nozzle, as the hose that comes with the handheld nozzle may not be long enough to easily move around the pALS.

Silicone Scrubbers

Both a silicone body brush with a long handle and a silicone handheld body scrubber were purchased to assist the pALS when he was still trying to shower himself. The cALS switched to a loofah and still utilized the silicone brushes during a period of time when the pALS went through an "itchy stage," trying to scrub the skin harder.

Washcloths

Investing in three dozen 100-percent cotton washcloths is highly recommended, as keeping the pALS clean and feeling their best is important. One dozen washcloths were a different color and reserved for use on the lower extremities of the body. The other two dozen were used for anything related to the face, such as washing, wiping the eyes, or wiping the mouth. Many washcloths were used each day.

Each day began with a warm washcloth to cleanse the eyes throughout all stages of ALS. As saliva production worsened, a second washcloth was used for wiping the mouth, cheeks and surrounding areas after cleaning the eyes.

Chapter 9

Toileting

A LOSS OF independence in the restroom may be realized by many early in the diagnosis; however, a bidet and a higher toilet may allow for some borrowed time with certain aspects in the restroom. The bidet will also add some height to the existing toilet, making it easier to stand without assistance.

The bidet was installed a few months after diagnosis, allowing the pALS to help himself until dressing became difficult. Initially, assistance was only needed to help pull clothing up. Shortly thereafter, help with handwashing in the sink and ensuring his hands were dry before walking with the rollator was also necessary. As time progressed, a gait belt was used to help the pALS stand from the toilet, prompting the decision to shop for and install a higher toilet. The higher toilet added just enough height to allow the pALS to stand on his own for a couple more months, before he again required assistance with the gait belt.

Bidet

There are many different brands and levels of bidets that can be purchased, from one with a few bells and whistles to many. Before purchasing a bidet, be mindful that you may have to have an electrical outlet installed in the bathroom, near the toilet, if there is not one existing, so that could be an added expense.

The bidet the pALS utilized was the BidetMate 3000 Series, which had some nice features, with one of the best for him being the handheld remote control. The pALS was able to utilize the remote control until late into middle-stage ALS, when assistance was needed.

Bucket

As the disease progressed, the pALS preferred using a five-gallon bucket with a plastic liner, suspended in the Hoyer lift sling, since bowel movements were not possible in a seated position. Although not ideal, this solution helped maintain bodily functions.

Commode Chair

The various shower/commode chairs tried are outlined in Chapter 8. Aside from the items previously mentioned, another important factor to consider when purchasing a commode chair is whether its height allows it to be placed over the toilet used by the pALS. In addition, check if there is enough space in the bathroom or water closet to maneuver the commode chair—with the pALS on it—into position.

Note: The "Shower Chair/Commode Chair, Reclining" we tried would not fit over any toilet taller than 15 inches, despite the chair's indicated height specifications. This was due to extra metal protruding on the underside of the chair, which prevented it from fitting over a higher toilet. The one from Nuprodx was too large to get into the water closet to try.

Disposable Gloves

Powder-free disposable gloves for the cALS to use, as needed.

Flushable Wipes

Flushable wipes were utilized from middle- to end-stage ALS, when the pALS could no longer use the bidet, as there was no way to get him into the water closet. The pALS preferred Cottonelle® Gentle Plus™ flushable wipes; however, any wipes can be used.

Incontinence Underwear

These were purchased proactively in the early part of middle-stage ALS in case the pALS attended an event and was unable to get out of his wheelchair to use the restroom. He wore them once to an event and never used them again; however, we had them on standby just in case.

Squatty Potty

This toilet stool came in handy after the higher toilet was purchased. Initially, cALS placed the pALS' feet on the stool for more stability. It was used only on occasion and not for very many weeks.

Toilet, High

Using a standard 17-inch toilet with an approximately 3-inch bidet was becoming a challenge for the pALS when rising from a seated position, so a 21-inch-high toilet was purchased. The added bidet height allowed the pALS to stand independently. When the pALS was unable to stand independently, the gait belt was used for assistance.

Urinal

This is a thick plastic men's bedpan bottle with a screw-on lid. As it became more difficult for the pALS to walk to the bathroom, a urinal started to be utilized, off and on, to lessen fatigue caused by walking. Eventually, the urinal was used exclusively while standing in front of the lift recliner. As the disease progressed, the Hoyer lift was required to utilize the urinal to empty the bladder. Since the pALS was getting into the Hoyer lift every 90 minutes to avoid pressure wounds, he was able to use the urinal frequently.

There are similar thick plastic portable women's bedpan bottles available, including ones that are specific for use in a hospital bed. I have no experience with female versions; however, it appears that many of these could be utilized with the Hoyer lift using a mesh toileting/shower sling, standing or in a lift recliner.

Chapter 10

Grooming

THE PALS SHOULD be treated like royalty as much as possible. ALS takes away life as it once was, and whatever can be done to make the pALS feel a little better should be done. Always feeling clean and groomed will not only make the pALS look better, but they will feel better all around; mentally and physically. Regular haircuts, shaving and nail trimming will make a world of difference in how the pALS looks and feels.

Cervical Neck Pillow

A different type of cervical neck pillow combined with a neck roll pillow was purchased for use when cutting the pALS' hair or shaving his face. The pillow had an indentation in the middle to accommodate the neck. The recliner lift chair had a headrest that flipped over the back of the chair. It was removed and the neck pillow inserted so the pALS could relax. This also made it easier to cut his hair since there was now room around the pillow that the chair headrest would not allow. This pillow was used during middle- through end-stage ALS.

Clippers, Hair

As the disease progresses, haircuts may become more of a challenge physically as well as financially. Initially, a stylist was coming to the home and cutting the pALS' hair. The pALS opted to start getting a buzz cut in middle-stage ALS, which was done at home by the cALS. His hair was cut about every 10 days until end-stage ALS, when it was done every four to six weeks.

Clippers, Nail

Nail clippers for the hands and toes will be necessary to keep the pALS' nails trimmed. After trimming, a nail file was used to get the nails a little shorter, for shaping and also to ensure no rough edges. Although not utilized with the pALS, there are electric nail trimmers available that may make the process easier and faster.

Hand Towel

This was moistened in water and heated in the microwave to make a hot, steamy towel for the face and neck before shaving. Shaving was done in a two-step process, first the neck and then the face, so the towel was applied two times, reheating in between. The towel was used when shaving with either a disposable or electric razor.

Nail File

A block-style nail file is useful when the pALS cannot use nail clippers. The block style makes it a little easier to hold, as it can be placed on a surface and held with the other hand, if needed. This was used by the pALS from early up to middle-stage ALS. After that point, a large emery board was used by the cALS to smooth the edges after nail clipping.

Razor, Disposable

Disposable razors are required for shaving the face and neck. A higher quality one for sensitive skin and a flexible blade may work better than some of the others.

Razor, Electric

An electric razor for shaving the face and neck—if affordable, one with a self-cleaning feature—makes it easier all around. The pALS preferred to be shaved with a disposable razor; however, he did not like the cALS' technique, so the electric razor was used most often.

Trimmer

A one-inch cordless electric trimmer is useful for touch-ups on any area that will make the pALS feel better. It can be used around the ears and back of the neck after a haircut, touch-up around the nose after shaving, on the eyebrows, arms, and more. It was also used to "knock-down" facial hair when it became too long to shave easily with an electric razor, or in late-stage ALS when the pALS did not feel like shaving as much, to shorten the facial hair without doing a full shave.

Trimmer, Ear and Nose

An electric ear and nose trimmer may be needed.

Chapter 11

Sleeping

SLEEPING WAS A constant challenge. From early- through end-stage ALS, the pALS spent most nights lying awake in bed, frustrated by the inability to sleep. In end-stage ALS, for approximately two weeks, the pALS napped during the day in the lift recliner, which provided some rest.

Getting comfortable became more difficult as the disease progressed, since severe anxiety caused his legs to stiffen and straighten throughout the night. At a minimum, we were up three times per hour trying to make adjustments and reposition the legs, although it was extremely difficult to get them to bend at the knees at times. During late- through end-stage ALS, the pALS had to sleep facing the nearest side of the bed due to claustrophobia. To change sides, the Hoyer lift was used to move across the bed and reposition him. The cALS slept in the same room with the pALS from middle- through end-stage ALS. In late-stage ALS when the California King adjustable bed was purchased, the cALS lay behind the pALS and always kept one hand on his side, due to the anxiety. If the pALS could not see or feel the cALS, he would have a panic attack. In addition, his ability to make noise had lessened and the cALS had to be close by to hear him over the music and noise app.

The pALS liked the temperature to be cold, so the house was generally kept at 63°F during the day and lowered to 60°F at night. The pre-cooling of the house would start approximately one hour before bedtime to ensure it was cool before going to bed.

The bedtime routine was adjusted as the disease progressed. It always consisted of the same steps; they were just done at different times or in different places, and anything that we could get done a little early, we would do, to shorten the bedtime preparation. For example, toothbrushing moved from the bathroom sink to the wheelchair, lift recliner, adjustable bed, and eventually back to the lift recliner. Once eating subsided, toothbrushing was not always done right at bedtime; it would be done earlier when possible. Medications too were adjusted to different times and places. Certain medications had a relaxing effect on the pALS, so those would have to be withheld from bedtime administration until we had actually gotten him into the bedroom or maybe even into bed, depending on the disease progression. Otherwise, depending on the stage, his legs could have become too relaxed to walk or even stand. Light sensitivity also became an issue, so overhead lights that were once kept on in the bedroom were off, and a lamp was used. Later, even the lamp was too much and would be turned off, so that just the lights from the bathroom were shining into the bedroom.

Toward the latter part of late-stage ALS, the bedtime routine would start in the lift recliner. The typical routine was as follows:

- Brush teeth and rinse with mouthwash
- Add Biofreeze patches to the hips
- Wipe eyes with a warm washcloth
- Use the suction device
- Get into the Hoyer lift and use the urinal
- Go to the bedroom and use the suction device
- Place pALS in bed on a pregnancy pillow, remove the sling, pull up and adjust underwear, tilt the bed to the sitting position, remove the pregnancy pillow and administer all medications.
- While the bed is going down, replace the pregnancy pillow and push the pALS up higher on the bed if needed. *Note: to push PALS, his knees were bent and cALS would hold his feet tightly while he assisted pushing.*
- Roll pALS onto his side, ensure pregnancy pillow is tucked under him in the back to stop him from rolling, ensure top arm is not

cutting off breath by moving onto pillow, adjust head and knees. Put a pillow between the knees. Pull the bottom arm up and out, and adjust the top arm to a comfortable position that is, again, not cutting off airflow.

- Adjust foot and head height on the bed, turn on the overhead fan, noise app, and music.
- Cover with a light covering.

The routine remained the same for end-stage ALS, except that medications were administered in the sling right after using the urinal, so there was no need to sit up in bed, nor to push him up higher. Oxygen was used some nights, so the nasal cannula was attached once the pALS was in the sleeping position and no pillow was inserted between the knees.

Bed, Adjustable Queen

The pALS went from a standard king-size bed to an adjustable queen-size bed, as the smaller size was more cost effective. This bed had a 14-inch, medium-soft mattress and the ability to tilt the head and foot areas upward. The bed was equipped with several additional features, including massage. The pALS opted for an adjustable bed rather than a hospital bed for comfort. Unfortunately, the pALS' height made the queen-size bed too short, especially since he was constantly sliding down. So, either the pALS' feet would hang off the bed, or the pALS would have to try to sleep at an angle to stay on the bed. Being unable to move and adjust made this a challenge. In addition, the mattress was too hard, causing additional hip pain over what the disease was already causing. The pALS could never get comfortable, so sleep was almost non-existent, aside from moving to the lift recliner in the morning and getting one to two hours of sleep there. This mattress was utilized for approximately nine months, from middle- to the beginning of late-stage ALS.

Bed, Adjustable California King

The pALS moved from a queen-size adjustable bed to a California King adjustable bed. Both beds had adjustable head and foot sections, but the California King offered a greater range of angles which proved to be beneficial. The mattress was 16 inches and ultra plush, so it was much softer than the other mattress. The bed was long enough that the pALS' feet did not hang off the end, even if he were to slide down a bit. With ALS, sleep is always a challenge. Although the new bed was more comfortable and the pALS spent a lot more time in it, he still wasn't completely comfortable or able to get the amount of sleep needed. This bed was used from late- to end-stage ALS.

Bed, Standard

A king-size bed with a soft mattress and a memory foam mattress topper had been purchased before the ALS diagnosis. It was used as long as possible by utilizing different pillows to prop up the pALS' head as needed. Sometimes, as many as nine pillows would be used in various positions around the pALS, as well as a pregnancy pillow.

Bed Ladder Assist Strap

This rope ladder ties to the footboard of the bed and has five hand grips. The premise is to help the pALS, who has limited upper body strength, sit up in bed and possibly scoot to the edge of the bed while holding on to the ladder. The physical therapist, who recommended this, also indicated it would help the pALS get into bed. The pALS tried this eight months after diagnosis, both while getting into bed and getting out of bed, but it was of no help and was never attempted again.

Biofreeze®

The pALS experienced a lot of hip pain in late- and end-stage ALS, which he described as more of a bone pain than muscle pain. No prescription narcotics seemed to relieve the pain, nor did he like narcotics, so we tried many different types of patches and creams. Biofreeze worked best for him. One patch was placed on each hip before bedtime each night. The roll-on gel was also used from time to time.

Getting Out of Bed

The pALS would propel himself upward by rolling back and forth to gain momentum, which worked into middle-stage ALS. Then the cALS started helping him sit up in bed and move to the side to sit. From there, the pALS was dressed and would use his rollator to get to his lift recliner. When the pALS could no longer walk that far, the rollator was used to stand and turn 45 degrees, so that the electric wheelchair could be moved up behind him to transport him to the lift recliner. Later into middle-stage ALS when the pALS was having more difficulty turning with the rollator, the Hoyer lift was used to get him in and out of bed, and dressing was done at the lift recliner.

Humidifier

Used with cool water to add moisture to the air at end-stage ALS.

Music

Music relaxed the pALS. The pALS' playlist was turned on each night (along with the noise app) to relax him and lessen anxiety. This was used during late- through end-stage ALS.

Noise App

The pALS could not rest without noise. An app with brown noise was turned on at a fairly high volume every night from early- through end-stage ALS.

Over-the-Counter Pain Relief

When the pALS experienced significant hip pain that prescription medications did not relieve, over-the-counter children's pain medications were explored, as they often come in liquid form. After receiving approval from the appropriate medical professionals, Children's Advil was added to the bedtime medications in late- and end-stage ALS. The pALS reported some relief with this medication.

Patient Turning Device

This is a U-shaped turning pillow with leg cutouts. The legs are strapped in, and it is supposed to assist in turning the pALS. It may work with someone closer to average height; it did not work at all with the pALS. The only thing that was turning was the pALS' legs, while the torso stayed in place. It was tried on one occasion and never again.

Pillow, Cervical

For neck pain relief, this device has a hollow design in the middle to provide support for back and side sleepers. The hollowed-out middle can be adjusted; however, it was still too short and did not provide any support for the pALS' neck. We tried several different brands of cervical pillows, but none of them worked. They were only tried in bed before going to sleep and could not be utilized for sleeping.

Pillow, King Size

Down alternative king-size pillows, 20 inches by 34 inches, were designed for back and side sleepers. Two were purchased to help elevate the pALS' head and try to make him more comfortable. These pillows did not do the trick; however, they later helped prop him on his side to prevent him from rolling onto his back. These were the first of many, many pillows purchased in search of the perfect pillow. We never found that, but we have a very large collection of pillows!

Pillow, Pregnancy

The *Momcozy* pregnancy pillow is U-shaped for full body, with a removable cover. This pillow was altered to make it more comfortable for the pALS. The longer side that goes in the front of the body was shortened substantially, so that it was slightly shorter than the back side and tied with a hair tie to secure it. A pillowcase was placed over this side and changed daily to ensure sanitary sleeping conditions for the pALS. Although the pALS did not find this pillow to be very comfortable after about six months, a satisfactory alternative pillow could not be found, and the pregnancy pillow continued to be used nightly through end-stage ALS.

Pillow, "Won't Go Flat"

This cotton and polyester king-size pillow provides firm support for neck and back sleepers. However, it was just another pillow that was not comfortable for the pALS and added to the pillow bone yard.

Pillow, Wedge

This large wedge pillow features a memory foam top, measuring 24 inches by 24 inches by 7.5 inches high. As with many pillows, this wedge pillow was tried once by the pALS and not used again. The pillow was quite large, provided substantial elevation of the head, and was not comfortable when lying on the back or side.

Supplement

Our pharmacist recommended melatonin to be taken with the sleeping pill to aid with sleeping. The pALS reported no difference in his ability to sleep; however, the supplement continued to be taken one hour before bedtime middle- through end-stage ALS.

Note: This is for information only and is not intended to prescribe or promote a supplement for other pALS.

Wedges

Two vinyl 45-degree bed wedges, though not used often, were used to try and alleviate hip and back pressure when lying on the side in bed. These were also experimented with in the lift recliner to remove pressure from the hips. They were used here and there from middle- to late-stage ALS.

Chapter 12

Living Room

MOST OF EACH day was spent in the living room, since this was part of the kitchen area and also housed the television and lift chair. There were six windows and a door with a window in the living room, three of which allowed the pALS to look outside from his lift chair. The first order of business each day was to open the blinds, so that when the pALS arrived in the living room, he could look outside. Initially, he would walk with his rollator each morning to the door with the window and look outside. When he could no longer do that, he would stand by his lift chair or sit in it and look outside. Some days he would declare, "It is a beautiful morning!"

When the pALS could no longer feed himself, all meals and snacks were eaten in the lift chair, utilizing the portable table described below.

Arm Table

A clip-on tray for the lift chair measuring 13 inches by 10.8 inches assisted as a place to put the television remote control and other things the pALS needed to reach when movement and hand dexterity were getting increasingly more difficult.

Blanket

A light blanket was required. As already mentioned, he liked the house to be kept cool, and his lift chair was located right under an air vent.

Although he was not always chilled, as the disease progressed, his knees and hands would turn purple if a light cover was not kept over them.

Cleaner, Device

With an AAC or a cellphone in the house, a premium cleaner for touchscreens will be needed. One with a microfiber cloth is recommended.

Cleaner, Eyeglass

If the pALS wears eyeglasses or sunglasses, a good quality cleaner and wiping cloth will be necessary.

Getting Up

When the pALS could walk using his rollator, he would get up once every hour and do laps up and down a long hallway, with the goal of a minimum of 10 laps each day. When he was no longer able to walk, he would get up and just stand, no less frequently than every 75 minutes. When the pALS opted to no longer stand in late-stage ALS due to hip pain, the Hoyer lift was used to get him up from his lift recliner every 90 minutes or earlier. We can say proudly that the pALS never developed a single pressure wound since he was not just left to sit or lie for a major portion of the day.

Hand Therapy, Rehabilitation Robot Glove

There are many of these rehabilitation robot gloves on the market, with different features and price points. The pALS always wanted to try one, and we researched them extensively. Although they are likely beneficial, there is a small investment required to purchase one or two of these. If the gloves do not work for anything else, they would at least help to keep the pALS' fingers and hands pliable and not so curled up and stiff.

Hand Therapy, Stress Balls

Stress squeeze balls come in three densities: soft, medium and hard. These were used in early-stage ALS to try and maintain motion and strength in both hands.

Headrest Protector

The lift recliner was made of cloth material, and the pALS' head would get hot and begin itching. A 17-inch by 27-inch non-slip leather headrest protector was placed on the headrest, which alleviated the itching. This was used from early- through end-stage ALS.

Hook and Loop Fastener

A small square of hook and loop fastener with adhesive was placed on a side table, with the other side being placed on the remote control, so the remote would not slide off the table when the pALS attempted to retrieve it. This was used in early-stage ALS.

Lift Chair Recliner

A lift recliner is a must for anyone with ALS. It made life easier in so many ways through all stages of ALS. The pALS was able to operate the chair himself through the early part of middle-stage ALS, if the remote was placed in a spot that he could reach on the chair, having limited mobility in his arms and hands. It allowed the pALS to sit and stand as long as possible on his own. When the pALS required assistance to stand, the lift recliner's ability to tilt forward significantly reduced the effort needed, making it easier than standing from a flat seated position. It was likely what enabled him to keep standing for as long as he did. It also made it very easy to get the split leg sling under the pALS, by performing the following steps:

- put the lift recliner in the forward position and lean the pALS forward, bending at the torso

- place the sling on the back of the pALS at the correct height and tuck the bottom of the sling, if possible

- put chair down to sitting position, pull sling and put around pALS' legs

- attach to the Hoyer lift and raise

Note: The pALS was above average height and he took a couple of weeks to research and find the perfect chair in early-stage ALS. In late-stage ALS, he was becoming uncomfortable in that chair, and we attempted to purchase two new chairs of different styles from the existing one, to replace it. Despite their dimensions being similar to the one he had, both chairs were way too small. In addition, the remotes that came with the chairs did not work the same way as the one on the existing chair, which would have made things more difficult. Lessons learned:

- *Despite the dimensions indicated on the chair, it may not fit the person, as one must be cognizant of the pALS' proportions, such as the torso to leg ratio.*

- *Chairs labeled for users above a specific height, are not necessarily based on the abovementioned proportional considerations.*

- *Remote controls are not created equal. Where the remote on his chair would lift the legs and recline the back at the same time—something really needed for a person who cannot control their body—other remotes/chairs we tried could only perform each of those functions separately.*

Lighter, Electric

The pALS utilized a rechargeable USB flameless electric candle lighter in early-stage ALS when a regular lighter was difficult to use; this enabled him to light candles nightly.

Portable Table

A universal swivel TV tray table came in handy. It had pre-drilled holes in the bottom, allowing a plastic cup holder to be attached. The pALS initially used the table to hold the remote control, drinking cups, or anything that needed to be within reach. As he transitioned to sippy cups, the drink holder could no longer be used and was removed. The cALS also used the tray table to hold food when the pALS was still able to eat, as he was fed while seated in his lift chair. After the feeding tube was in place, the table held medications, water, food, supplements, and other items taken orally or given through the tube. This table was used daily from early- through end-stage ALS.

Pressure Relieving Cushion

A PURAP® liquid, air, and foam wheelchair cushion was acquired in middle-stage ALS to replace both the ROHO and *CG Air* cushions that the pALS was using in the recliner lift chair for comfort. Many other pads had been tried prior to this, and the pALS reported that this was the most comfortable of all pads. The drawback at the time was that the pALS could still stand, and the cushion was very thin, making it more difficult for him to get into a standing position. In addition, the thinner cushion made him sit lower in the chair, making the seam at the bottom of the headrest press uncomfortably into his back. The *CG Air* cushion provided the extra height needed to be able to get up to a standing position and eliminate the discomfort on his back, so the PURAP cushion was no longer used, and the *CG Air* cushion was used through end-stage ALS.

Remote Control Hooks

A plastic wall hook holder with self-adhesive was tried out on a side table to make the remote control easier for the pALS to retrieve; however, the pALS could not put the remote control on the hook.

ROHO Mosaic Cushion

Originally purchased for the lift recliner, it was also used in the wheelchair, as the seat that came with the wheelchair was extremely hard and uncomfortable. The ROHO was used mostly during middle-stage ALS. For a short time, the pALS' heels were placed on the cushion as well, as a way of trying to relieve some of the pain and pressure on his heels while in the lift chair.

Slippers

Microsuede moccasin memory foam house shoes with hard soles helped to keep the pALS warm and comfortable in winter. The hard soles also provided stability, helping him walk when balance was getting harder.

Chapter 13

Relaxation

We did whatever we could to help the pALS relax, especially in late- and end-stage ALS when anxiety, claustrophobia, and panic attacks became more pronounced. Although claustrophobia was present throughout all stages of ALS, it worsened dramatically overnight and never improved. Anxiety began in late-stage ALS and got progressively worse. The pALS would experience a panic attack if the cALS was not within sight. Visitors were limited to those who were calm and free of stress or nervousness, as the pALS could sense these emotions, which would in turn heighten his anxiety.

Acupressure Mat and Pillow Set

A cushioned mat and pillow with lots of plastic spikes on the mat and pillow were supposed to provide pain relief. Hoping for some pain relief in the neck, the pALS tried the pillow while sitting in the lift recliner one time. It did not help, and laying the neck on the pillow was painful.

Candles

The pALS loved candles, and one was lit every night until late-stage ALS, when he no longer wanted them burning. Candles brought him a sense of relaxation, and he enjoyed choosing the evening's scent.

Massage, Eye

This rechargeable eye mask massager goes over the eyes and straps around the back of the head. It had Bluetooth® so that the pALS' music could be played while the massage was taking place. This was used during middle-stage ALS, prior to the extreme claustrophobia, and he enjoyed it thoroughly, along with the simultaneous foot rub. It is also a nice relaxation tool for the cALS.

Massage, Foot

Manual foot massage: The pALS went from having ticklish feet to asking for a foot massage every day. An electric foot and calf massager was purchased, and like many other things, was tried once and never used again. He preferred the manual massage, and it turned out to be one of the only ways to relax him once the major anxiety and panic attacks started. This was part of our daily routine from middle- through end-stage ALS, taking place throughout the day and always at night, shortly before the bedtime routine started, in an effort to relax the pALS.

Massage, Head and Scalp

A manual head and scalp massager with twenty metal fingers was used to help the pALS rest, relax, and reduce anxiety from middle- to late-stage ALS. In late- and end-stage ALS, he preferred a head rub with the hands instead.

Massage, Neck

The pALS required a daily massage of the neck and shoulder area using just the hands, as he had extreme neck pain from degenerating discs. This was done from early-stage ALS through the first part of late-stage ALS. Initially, it provided a lot of relief for the degenerating discs; however, as the disease progressed, it became quite uncomfortable for the pALS to have the neck area massaged.

Massage, Percussion Gun

A percussion gun massager was used occasionally in early- and middle-stage ALS on the upper back and neck area mostly. It was also used on the thigh and calf area when needed. As the disease progressed and muscles became tight and sore in late- and end-stage ALS, it was used more frequently. In late-stage ALS, it was used mostly on the legs, especially the calf muscles and hips. In end-stage ALS, the gluteal and hip muscles were the main focus. The easiest way to do the gluteal muscles was while the pALS was in the Hoyer lift. This was easily accomplished during the "standing" intervals every 90 minutes.

Massage, Professional

If the budget allows, including professional massage therapy in the routine for both pALS and cALS is beneficial. When the pALS is no longer able to travel to the massage therapist and/or lie on the stomach, a mobile massage therapist may be available for home visits. The pALS had a massage therapist recommended by the OT, who would come over and perform the massage while the pALS reclined or sat in the recliner lift chair. This was done mostly in middle-stage ALS and a few times in late-stage ALS. When anxiety and claustrophobia heightened, it was no longer relaxing to get a massage.

Massage, Transcutaneous Electrical Nerve Stimulation (TENS)

A TENS massager sends electrical impulses through adhesive pads placed on the skin over a specific area and offers numerous settings. The pALS thought it might be beneficial and relaxing for the cALS to use. The cALS used it once and found it acceptable. On one occasion, the adhesive pads were placed on the pALS' neck area during middle-stage ALS. While the pALS did not dislike the experience, he enjoyed the manual massage more, so the TENS was never used again.

Headphones or Earbuds

The pALS loved music and liked to listen to it at a high volume at times. The headphones and earbuds allowed him to do so. The earbuds were also beneficial during middle-stage ALS, when the pALS would attempt to sleep in his lift recliner in the mornings; the earbuds plus the sleeping mask would usually be the recipe for his getting a little bit of sleep.

Music

Music helped in relaxation throughout all stages of ALS and was especially beneficial in the late- and end-stages for relieving anxiety.

Range of Motion Exercises

Range of motion exercises are so important and can make a world of difference in how the pALS feels. If able, the pALS can move around and try to maintain a range of motion in the limbs a few times each day. In our case, while still mobile, the pALS would do laps daily around the house with his rollator, lift and lower his legs while sitting, stretch his legs back as far as possible, rotate his arms, and more. As the disease progressed and the pALS was not able to do the movements on his own or do them to the extent previously done, the cALS took over. The exercises were performed daily on all upper and lower body extremities, from shoulders to toes through end-stage ALS. Working the legs would make the pALS feel fatigued, so the goal was to complete the lower body as early as possible in the day and the arms anytime thereafter. The entire body was generally not done at one time, to ensure that the pALS did not get too tired.

Spa/Hot Tub

The pALS was having quite a bit of hip pain and would opt to stay inside the house in late- and end-stage ALS. During end-stage ALS, an inflatable spa was purchased, which was fairly inexpensive compared to other spas. We needed a way to get the pALS into the spa with the Hoyer lift. Utilizing the pALS' creativity on a limited budget, a platform was built out of four pallets and two pieces of plywood, allowing the Hoyer lift to be driven underneath the spa so the pALS could be put inside.

The spa was a big hit with the pALS; the only thing he did not like was that he floated while in the sling. A scuba belt and weights were purchased to hold the pALS down. Unfortunately, we only got to try this method once, and the belt was just laid on the lap of the pALS, so it did not work. Afterwards, the pALS said the belt should have been put on properly, and it would have been effective in holding him down.

Also, as part of the spa, there was a bath pillow placed on the side for the pALS to rest his head and neck and a floating Bluetooth speaker to connect to his favorite music from the Tobii Dynavox.

Chapter 14

Travel

THE FINAL TIME the pALS traveled was during middle-stage ALS. Both air and train travel were explored, as there was concern about taking the electric wheelchair on the airplane and risking damage. It was also assumed that train travel would be more cost effective than air travel; that assumption was not accurate.

Having determined that air travel was the fastest and least costly option, we reached out to the ALS Association at the destination and were able to borrow an electric wheelchair, shower/commode chair, Hoyer lift, rollator, and portable ramp. Logistically, more effort was required due to not having the personal electric wheelchair at the airport; however, there was peace of mind knowing that the pALS' own wheelchair was not potentially getting damaged on the airplane. Since additional time is needed at the airport, it's important to arrive earlier than usual—everything takes longer, including getting through security and settling into the airplane seat. From the curbside, the pALS was transferred from his wheelchair to one owned by the airline. His personal wheelchair was then placed back into his vehicle and parked in the parking structure so it would be there upon our return. The airline was able to assist with transporting him to/from the airplane.

Prior to traveling, if neck control is an issue, it's important to find a way to support the neck during the flight, prior to arriving at the airport. Based on information from the airline regarding the seat's recline, it seemed the seat would tilt far enough to help keep the head back. However, that was not the case, and the travel pillow was not strong enough to hold the neck, nor was the universal neck brace or Headmaster Collar. The cALS ended up stabilizing the pALS' head the entire flight. For the return trip, a family member rigged up a head strap that would go around the seat, but the pALS chose not to try it.

Some other things to consider before heading out on a trip include the types of activities in which the pALS may be participating. Are there beaches, and if so, is there accessibility to the sand? Are rental beach wheelchairs available? Are there parks with paved, wheelchair-friendly trails? Do any of these activities or rentals require advance reservations?

Authorization Letter

Prior to any travel, check with the neurologist to ensure that travel is permitted. In addition, request a letter from the neurologist stating that the pALS is under the neurologist's care, including the diagnosis and the neurologist's contact information. Keep the letter with the pALS at all times, so that in the event medical attention becomes necessary, it can be presented to the available medical personnel.

Beach Wheelchair

A beach wheelchair has large tires designed to roll over sand. Both manual and motorized models are available, and some beaches also offer amphibious wheelchairs that can float in the water. Since availability varies and not all beaches provide them, it is important to research options before leaving on a trip.

Blankets

Airline blankets help keep the pALS comfortable during the flight and can be used to brace the hands, support the back, and help the pALS stay more upright. On the return flight, we used nine folded blankets to stabilize him as much as possible.

Call Ahead

To make prior accessibility arrangements, airlines require information regarding whether a personal wheelchair will be included in the travel or not. If so, the airline must be notified of its dimensions, and they must approve whether or not there is space in the cargo area. Some airlines also require forms to be completed for the wheelchair. In addition, extra assistance must be requested for the pALS, and this can be pre-arranged during the same phone call.

Tip: Prior to the flight, call the airline again to ensure that the pre-arrangements that were made are in fact noted in the system and that staff will be available to help. Our experience was that nothing was noted in the system for the first flight, and on the return flight, even after verifying that assistance would be available, little help was provided, with virtually no empathy for our situation. Thankfully, there was a physical therapist as a passenger on the first flight who was willing to lend a helping hand before, during and after the flight.

Direct Flight

Book a direct flight. If no direct flight is available, book the shortest duration of travel available, including layovers, and change planes as few times as possible.

EarPlanes®

These assist in relieving any pain or pressure in the ears while flying. The pALS did not care for these; however, the cALS found them useful.

External Catheter

Condom catheters are available for both men and women. This was utilized for air travel in case the pALS needed to use the restroom, as there was no way to do so on the airplane when traveling with middle-stage ALS. The catheters were self-sealing and came with a leg bag, which straps around the leg with an adjustable strap and tubing long enough to reach the ankle of an above-average height individual. The bag can be emptied via a valve at the bottom, if needed. It is a good idea to take along an empty bottle in case the catheter needs to be emptied during the flight.

First Class Seating

If the budget permits, there is more leg room in first class and fewer seats per row, allowing a row for just the pALS and cALS. In addition, the seats recline farther than in the economy class, though not far enough to assist with head control. If the pALS has difficulty with head control, the head will still fall forward in these seats.

Hotel

When booking a hotel room, an assumption is that an ADA room comes equipped with a roll-in shower. Unfortunately, this is not always the case and needs to be verified with the hotel. In addition, if a Hoyer lift is going to be utilized, ensure there is enough room for the lift to be moved around and that there are no obstacles under the bed that will prevent the lift from sliding under. Many hotels have wooden bases underneath the beds that will not allow a Hoyer lift to be utilized.

Liquid Nutrition

The basic rule with airline travel is that larger amounts of liquid cannot go through security. It is okay to carry liquid nutrition along, if the security personnel are informed of the liquid when arriving at the security checkpoint. It will be inspected and allowed through.

Pillows

Airline pillows are another way to stabilize the pALS and keep them from moving from side to side. The pillows do not, however, assist with keeping the pALS from slipping off the seat.

Rental Vehicle

When renting an ADA vehicle for ground transportation, call ahead and make arrangements before arriving at the destination. Ideally, see if someone can meet you at the airport with the vehicle and borrowed wheelchair.

Rollator

When the pALS first began using a rollator, he traveled once by air. The airline provided extra assistance to the gate with a wheelchair and the rollator was checked at the gate. Unfortunately, one of the screws holding the rollator together was lost in transit, presenting an issue with being able to use the rollator without it falling apart. Be mindful that this is a possibility and either go prepared with extra parts or have an alternative plan in mind, should this occur.

ROHO Mosaic Cushion

The cushion that was used at home in the lift recliner and wheelchair was also placed in the airplane seat to make it more comfortable for the pALS.

Sleep Mask

A dark cloth mask with a head strap was used for sleeping during travel in early-stage ALS and when sleeping in a room without room-darkening curtains when not traveling.

Suitcase

Depending on disease progression, there may be a lot of equipment that must be packed. Aside from packing as early as possible to avoid undue stress on the day of the trip, take just one large suitcase if possible for both the pALS and the cALS. However, this may not be possible with all of the equipment that needs to be carried.

Toiletry Bag

Clear quart-size bags with zippers come in a set of three. The bags are intended for women's make-up. For travel, these are perfect for packing and storing enteral supplies, such as extension tubes and syringes.

Train Travel

As expected, train travel generally takes longer than air travel. When researching, there are several items to explore, such as how many hours or days it will take for a one-way and a round trip. This adds stress to the pALS and may take days out of the enjoyable part of the trip and/or add to the overall timeline.

If traveling overnight, is an ADA room required? Is just the room needed or an ADA room with a restroom? As we learned, only certain trains have these rooms, and they run on specific routes. In order to reserve one of these rooms, an extra day was added to our already long trip, as the train's route was far out of the way of our planned destination. Another consideration could be whether there is a train station close to the origin and the destination. If so, does one of the ADA-compliant trains travel through those destinations? On both ends, we had to travel a considerable distance to/from the train station. This made the logistics even harder, since we were being met with the rental van and wheelchair at our destination.

Travel Pillow

A memory foam neck pillow specifically for travel that was soft and breathable was used for travel during early-stage ALS. It was attempted the last time the pALS traveled, too; however, it could not hold the head.

Chapter 15

Daily Schedule

THIS IS A brief rundown of a typical day during middle- through end-stage ALS. It does not include every detail, just some major ones. As always, there are many moving parts involved, so everything is not done at the same time every day and not necessarily in the same order. Depending on the day and how much the pALS' is able to assist, the morning routine may take several hours. As eating becomes more difficult, it adds a lot of time to the schedule.

Middle-Stage ALS

The pALS had a lot of appointments, both in-person and with home health. Range of motion exercises were done by occupational therapy twice per week and physical therapy two to three times per week. The cALS would help work the muscles the therapist didn't focus on that day.

Morning

- Sit up and get dressed on the side of the bed, transfer to the wheelchair using a rollator
- Use the restroom, brush teeth and wipe eyes with a warm washcloth
- Take morning medications
- Have breakfast and coffee
- Take vitamins

- Take a walk outside in the wheelchair
- Range of motion exercises for the lower body
- Have a smoothie
- Stand every 60 – 75 minutes and move around and stretch as much as possible in lift recliner

Afternoon

- Eat lunch
- Range of motion exercises for the upper body
- Take medications
- Head massage
- Eat snack
- Stand every 60 – 75 minutes and move around, and stretch as much as possible in the lift recliner

Evening

- Eat dinner
- Take medications
- Shave face (every two days)
- Shower, wash hair, clean feeding tube
- Stand every 60 – 75 minutes and move around and stretch as much as possible in the lift recliner

Night

- Stand every 60 – 75 minutes and move around and stretch as much as possible in the lift recliner
- Eat snack
- Take medications
- Relaxation and massage
- Transfer from lift recliner to wheelchair to bed using rollator
- Go to bed, roll onto side, adjust body for comfort
- Listen to the noise app

Late-Stage ALS

The pALS only had physical therapy one day per week and very few other appointments. Saliva was very heavy, requiring constant suctioning, and anxiety and panic attacks also started; all of this took up a lot of time throughout the day.

Morning

- Get out of bed with the Hoyer lift and use the urinal
- Go to the lift recliner, apply deodorant and dress
- Wipe eyes and mouth with warm washcloths
- Liquid breakfast, snacks and water
- Take morning medications and vitamins
- Clean the inside of the nose
- Foot and/or head massage
- Range of motion exercises for the lower body
- Get up in the Hoyer lift and use the urinal every 90 minutes or less

Afternoon

- Liquid lunch, snacks and water
- Range of motion exercises for the upper body
- More medications
- Shave face (every three days)
- Shower and wash hair (every other day)
- Wash face and clean feeding tube
- Get up in the Hoyer lift and use the urinal every 90 minutes or less
- Clean the inside of the nose
- Foot massage

Evening

- Liquid dinner, snacks and water
- More medications

- Relaxation and massage
- Get up in the Hoyer lift and use the urinal every 90 minutes or less

Night

- Get up in the Hoyer lift and use the urinal every 90 minutes or less
- More medications
- Foot and head massage
- Go to bed, roll onto side, adjust body for comfort
- Listen to the noise app and music

End-Stage ALS

Saliva was still heavy, requiring frequent suctioning, but not as much as previously needed. The panic attacks were less frequent; however, anxiety levels were very high.

Morning

- Get out of bed and use the urinal
- Go to the lift recliner, apply deodorant and dress
- Wipe eyes and mouth with warm washcloths
- Liquid breakfast, snacks and water
- Take morning medications and vitamins
- Clean the inside of the nose
- Foot and/or head massage
- Range of motion exercises for the lower body
- Get up in the Hoyer lift and use the urinal every 90 minutes

Afternoon

- Liquid lunch, snacks and water
- Range of motion exercises for the upper body
- More medications
- Spa/Hot Tub
- Shave face (every four to five days)

- Shower and wash hair (every two to three days)
- Wash face and clean feeding tube
- Wipe down body with soap and water (when not showering)
- Get up in the Hoyer lift and use the urinal every 90 minutes
- Clean the inside of the nose
- Foot massage

Evening

- Liquid dinner, snacks and water
- More medications
- Relaxation and massage
- Get up in the Hoyer lift and use the urinal every 90 minutes

Night

- Get up in the Hoyer lift and use the urinal every 90 minutes
- More medications
- Foot and head massage
- Go to bed, roll onto side, adjust body for comfort
- Listen to the noise app and music

Chapter 16

Medical and Later Stage Planning

SOME INSURANCE COMPANIES allow more flexibility than others; however, the pALS will likely have the ability to shop around and find the perfect medical doctor, neurologist, palliative care, hospice, etc. Some organizations, including ALS support groups and other pALS who have been navigating the system, can assist in this. Be mindful too that there may be a hospital or medical center in your area that provides funding if the pALS submits a grant application. The funding is generally provided for six months at a time, after which re-application is required, and it will cover at least a percentage or potentially even all of the pALS' co-pay for services rendered at their facility.

Hospice

There may come a time when hospice enters the discussions. This again is something that is a personal choice and is not required for the pALS. Not all hospice agencies are created equal, and you are not required to use the one recommended by a medical or palliative care professional. Hospice agencies do not all allow the same things regarding medications, nutrition, machines, and other services, so it is wise to shop around if this is important to the pALS. When deciding, consider the following:

- Interview multiple hospice agencies within your region to determine which is the best fit, ensuring the pALS is involved in each interview, if able.

- Allow the pALS to meet with agency nurses to check the level of comfort.
- Will the pALS be better served staying with home health or transitioning to hospice?
- Consider the financial aspect in terms of staying with home health versus hospice.
- Is in-home or inpatient hospice a better fit?

Allow the pALS to make the decision on whether or not to proceed with hospice care. If proceeding, and able, the pALS should be allowed to make the choice on which hospice and the date on which to begin. Hospice is an extremely difficult decision, and no pressure should be put on the pALS to move forward with hospice care.

Note: It may be likely that a referral will have to be requested for each hospice that you want to interview. This is standard and does not tie you in with the hospice; it just allows the hospice to speak with you. Ensure you have a list of all medications, including dosage, available to share with the hospice, as well as a list of machines, including the models and frequency of use. If all medications and machines are documented by the medical professional making the referral, those can be forwarded to the hospice and save some legwork on your end.

Neurologist

Based on experience as well as word of mouth, a lot of neurologists out there do not understand ALS and many lack compassion. Some are absolutely fantastic as well. Depending on which scenario rings true in your case, this may be another area where the pALS will want to do some research and shop around. Short of naming some exemplary neurologists, a starting point may be looking at hospitals or facilities that are heavily involved in ALS research or getting enrolled with *Synapticure* and starting there.

This is another area where the pALS must feel comfortable, as there will be a lot of interaction with the neurologist. It will be obvious within the first few visits whether or not the neurologist shows empathy and that the pALS' best interest is in mind when making decisions and navigating ALS. Following are some things to consider when evaluating a neurologist.

Does the neurologist:

- demonstrate knowledge and experience in managing ALS?
- order genetic testing shortly after diagnosis?
- discuss available ALS medications?
- mention or discuss clinical trials that may be available?
- respond to inquiries outside of appointments and/or in a timely manner?

More considerations:

- Does the pALS feel comfortable with the neurologist, the given diagnosis and that all possible testing has been completed?

After the initial diagnosis, it is still possible to work with another neurologist. Do not feel like you are stuck with the one who diagnosed the pALS, if a few months down the road, it is not feeling like a good fit. It is never too late to switch or talk to another health professional.

Palliative Care

There may come a time when a neurologist says there is nothing more that they can do for the pALS and makes a referral to palliative care. This is again a personal choice and not required. The benefit is that the pALS can get immediate prescriptions for pain, if needed, rather than potentially waiting for a doctor or neurologist to respond and prescribe. There are palliative care nurses that come to the home as well as palliative care that requires travel to a facility. As with most services, palliative care visits may come with co-pay or out-of-pocket costs.

Primary Care Physician

The pALS may continue seeing a primary care physician (PCP) at least once per year for insurance renewal requirements, bloodwork, and general check-ups, particularly during early- and into middle-stage ALS. The PCP will likely be the one who orders home health, including speech therapy, occupational therapy, physical therapy and nursing.

Note: In our case, the pALS' palliative care recommended bringing primary care into the home. This seemed like a good idea, since travel was becoming increasingly difficult for the pALS. However, our experience with this was not positive. The pALS requested a medical doctor (MD), and although promised there would be one who would come out, this turned out not to be an option for a home visit. It was generally a nurse practitioner (NP), of which we already had many, through palliative care and various other medical offices. Although requiring few visits to a PCP at that point of the disease, the in-home PCP made several visits per month. Most of the cost had to be paid out-of-pocket, and the NPs that were coming over had no familiarity with ALS at all. This led to the NP going back to the office to speak to the MD and then making a call to update us; all of this extra was an additional charge on top of the visit. In addition, none of the information passed down was useful at all, leaving any concerns we had about things occurring with the pALS unanswered and sometimes forcing us to reach out to the original PCP for assistance.

Chapter 17

Organizations

ORGANIZATIONS LISTED IN this section are resources that may be explored for assistance, including borrowing equipment, obtaining grants, healthcare, nutrition, scholarships, and ALS education or support. This list is not comprehensive and does not capture all available resources, nor all the valuable services each organization may provide. There are many resources, though some are regional and only available to residents of a specific area. Check your local community to see what may be available to you.

The ALS Association

They have many resources available, such as grants, loaned durable medical equipment, clinics, and more. Check your local chapter to see the services provided in your area.

ALS United®

Each affiliate offers a unique mix of services, shaped by its budget, local partnerships, and community needs. Nearly all affiliates provide support groups, care navigation, and loaned durable medical equipment.

Augie's Quest

The organization is dedicated to finding cures and treatments for pALS and aims to enhance patient care and support services. They raise funds and awareness for cutting-edge research and fast-track effective treatments.

I AM ALS®

This group advocates for ALS and provides support, resources, and education for pALS and their families; they started Synapticure.

Live Like LOU Foundation

Provides support to ALS families, such as volunteers to assist around the home, grants for respite and home improvement, financial assistance for children in ALS families for higher education, and ALS awareness.

Oley Foundation

This non-profit foundation provides many services related to home nutrition support. Individuals post unneeded enteral supplies on this foundation's website that others in need can obtain. The person seeking the supplies just pays postage, not for the supplies. We acquired many cases of liquid nutrition by going through this website, prior to insurance approving the purchase of nutrition for the pALS.

Sean M. Healey & AMG Center for ALS

Working to discover life-saving therapies for pALS, this is a resource for clinical trials as well as patient and family support and education.

Synapticure

This institution provides accessible care to patients and caregivers, offering virtual neurology and behavioral health care to all states within the United States. They may assist with genetic testing as well. Care coordinators can assist with durable medical equipment and other healthcare needs to remove some of the burden that comes along with those decisions.

Team Gleason

This organization empowers families to gain access to available technologies and alternative mobility. They may be able to assist with grants for things such as communication devices, a wheelchair seat elevator, respite care in certain areas or even a travel adventure.

Chapter 18

Supporting the Caregiver

SELF-CARE IS VERY important for the cALS. Many cALS not only care for the pALS 24/7, but are also responsible for keeping the household running and completing all inside and outside chores. The cALS should do anything enjoyable, whether it is meditating, yoga, going for a walk outdoors, getting a haircut or massage, gardening, going to the gym, or shopping, to name a few. Although going away from the house may not be completely relaxing, if the pALS does not have anyone sitting with them, it is still beneficial for the cALS to get away.

In our case, we experienced both the benefits and the challenges of this balance. The pALS always put others before himself. He would ask to be situated in his lift recliner and consistently encouraged the cALS to take a break of at least one hour per day, while it was still possible. He knew the disease would eventually progress to a point where he could no longer be left alone. The pALS' disease progressed very quickly, and after six months, taking a break for any length of time was close to impossible. Fortunately, the pALS had an amazing home health nurse. The nurse would watch a comedy show with the pALS, on her own time, one hour per week, to give the cALS a break. This could only be done for a couple of months, until the pALS' anxiety got so bad that the cALS could not be away from him for more than a few minutes at a time. Even then, his nurse still came by for comedy hour and we would all watch together, giving the cALS a chance to rest.

When breaks away from the house were no longer possible, there were still ways to find renewal together. Even short walks or time outside with the pALS proved rejuvenating. If a spa or hot tub is available, that is quite relaxing to do together as well. Although we didn't get the spa until end-stage ALS, it gave the pALS something to look forward to every day, and it really helped the mental well-being of both the pALS and cALS to be outside of the house.

In late-stage ALS, the pALS surprised the cALS with some foot soak, consisting of Epsom and sea salt. Breaks were difficult at this point due to the pALS' saliva production and anxiety attacks. Whenever possible, the cALS would take a 15-minute break in the evening to do a foot soak. That break was much appreciated and was rejuvenating as well.

Another helpful item that the pALS got for the cALS was reusable gel finger cots by Pnrskter®. Along with liquid bandage, these cushioned covers reduced discomfort and were beneficial in helping to heal split fingers from excessive handwashing. In addition to that purpose, the pALS thought they might prevent the cALS' fingers from getting pinched on the Hoyer lift. It was difficult to work with the pALS while wearing the finger cots, especially when the cALS had to grip clothing and other things; however, they were perfect to use when the pALS was in bed.

It is also important that the cALS eat right to maintain overall health and strength. As the pALS requires more care, it becomes harder for the cALS to find time for a meal, especially during what may be considered a typical mealtime. When there is some extra time available while the pALS is relaxing, doing some food preparation will help. For example, prepare several jar salads with your favorite healthy ingredients—such as olive oil, black pepper and chili flakes to taste, plus a handful of cucumbers, nuts like walnuts or almonds, red onion, corn and tomatoes with either romaine lettuce or spinach. Cooking meat in advance for a few days at a time and keeping a variety of frozen vegetables on hand makes for a quick meal. It is also a good idea to have fruit and nuts available for snacks between meals.

Something to be mindful of is that cooking food or sitting next to the pALS to eat may increase saliva production. So, eating cold foods like sandwiches and smoothies may be something to consider, and if anything needs to be cooked, do it when the pALS is not in the room and air the kitchen out afterwards to get rid of the smell. That way, the warm food can simply be reheated in the microwave or air fryer for a short time, and the smell will not be as strong as with a freshly-cooked meal.

Beyond food preparation, if there is anything that can lighten the cALS' load, it is worth exploring. One example is ordering groceries online for delivery. This option can be helpful through all stages of ALS, and while able, the pALS can even assist with the ordering process. Some grocery stores will also deliver medications, provided they are not narcotics.

In addition to services, outside resources and people can make a huge difference too. If friends, neighbors, or community resources offer help, it is important to say yes. Even if it feels manageable on your own, accepting support can ease the cALS' burden and make daily life feel less overwhelming. It also reassures the pALS, who may otherwise feel guilty or helpless, to know the weight is not falling solely on the cALS. In our case, the pALS had a close buddy whose entire family supported us immensely pitching in with house chores, repairs, and errands, especially during late- and end-stage ALS. This support was invaluable, helping us keep up with countless tasks that otherwise would have been left undone.

Chapter 19

Closing Word for Family and Friends

ALS IS A disease that robs friends and family members of their lives, and some more quickly than others. Every day is a fight for that individual; a fight to take just one more step, a fight to scratch that itch, a fight to see another day.

Your loved one may no longer be able to have the same kind of conversation as in the past, take that run, go to dinner, go fishing or drink a beer with you, but that person is still the same person mentally. It is still the same person with whom you once enjoyed spending time; it's just that their body is failing.

Having a fatal disease can become very lonely for a pALS, especially when confined to a chair or maybe a bed. The mental anguish of knowing one's fate is depressing; knowing that they may never see their kids grow up, knowing that they have so much life left to live yet are unable to do so. A pALS has a hard time turning off their thoughts, knowing what the future holds. Many friends and family members who were once close seem to have disappeared, and few reach out or ever ask how the pALS is doing.

Currently, there is nothing that can be done to save the person's life; however, the life that is left to live can be made as enjoyable as possible. Despite having a fatal disease, a pALS does want to be asked how they are doing, feel loved and cared for, spend social time with friends and family and feel "normal" again.

As the disease progresses, everything may feel overwhelming; it may feel as if there just aren't enough hours in the day to get things done. Take a deep breath. Everything will get done, it just may not be within the timeline you desire. The laundry will eventually get folded and put away, even if it is one shirt here and there. The bed may or may not get made, and the house may not get picked up or cleaned. It will happen eventually, even if it is just good enough and not totally to your standards. All of this is minor compared to what the pALS is dealing with and facing.

One of the most important things to always remember is to be kind and treat the pALS like a king or queen. The pALS would give anything to be the one who is not facing a fatal disease. The pALS would rather be going to work every day. The pALS would rather be the cALS. The pALS would take anything that is thrown their way not to be sick.

Hopefully, this guide will help in navigating through the journey with ALS and provide information that will assist in making both pALS' and cALS' days a little easier and maybe a little brighter. As Brian used to say, "I try to start every day positively. Every day is a new day, and whatever happened yesterday is gone and in the past. I don't have time for negativity in what is left of my short life. It took me getting a fatal disease to see this." So please be mindful of Brian's words; put a big smile on your face each morning when you awaken; and remember, you are not alone in this fight.

www.ingramcontent.com/pod-product-compliance
Lightning Source LLC
Chambersburg PA
CBHW032056040426
42335CB00036B/422